Solutions to Access Safe and Drinking Water in Africa

Solutions to Access Safe and Drinking Water in Africa

Editors
Mammo Muchie and *Angathevar Baskaran*

AFRICA WORLD PRESS
TRENTON | LONDON | CAPE TOWN | NAIROBI | ADDIS ABABA | ASMARA | IBADAN | NEW DELHI

AFRICA WORLD PRESS
541 West Ingham Avenue | Suite B
Trenton, New Jersey 08638

Book design: Dawid Kahts
Cover art: Ananthy Baskaran

Library of Congress Cataloging-in-Publication Data:

Names: Muchie, Mammo, editor. | Baskaran, Angathevar, editor.
Title: Solutions to access safe and drinking water in Africa / editors, Mammo Muchie and Angathevar Baskaran.
Description: Trenton : Africa World Press, 2017. | Includes bibliographical references and index.
Identifiers: LCCN 2017008499| ISBN 9781569025611 (hb : alk. paper) | ISBN 9781569025628 (pb : alk. paper)
Subjects: LCSH: Water resources development--Africa. | Water quality management--Africa. | Water-supply--Africa. | Sanitation--Africa.
Classification: LCC TD315 .S65 2017 | DDC 333.9115096--dc23
LC record available at https://lccn.loc.gov/2017008499

This book is dedicated to

All those children and women across Africa who have to trek miles and miles to fetch water for every day survival

Contents

Preface

Access to Water is a Human Right

Mammo Muchie & Angathevar Baskaran

The contributions to this book originating from research papers mainly but not exclusively from various issues of the Journal of Science, Technology, Innovation and Development (AJSTID) reveal and feature the shared concern of researchers determined to discover new knowledge and insights on water issues that are pertinent in Africa. Clean water on the tap is still a luxury in Africa. Water exists in abundance but not in ways it can be accessed and used readily by ordinary people. The millennium development goals aimed at halving by 2015 the proportion of the population without sustainable access to safe drinking water and basic sanitation. Nevertheless, safe drinking water to all the rural households in Africa and safe water supply to all the people of Africa remain still a big challenge. Water is more critical than electricity and other necessities in life. One can find a way to live without electricity, but life without water is inconceivable. The priority to get water clean and accessible to all at the same time brooks no delay. This book addresses various ways of how clean water production can be generated. We have put together contributions by various authors that used a combination of primary and secondary data to generate new and original insights to advance knowledge in the area of water studies related to Africa.

The central concept that provides the organizing principle of all the contributions in this book is undertaking very specfic research to discover the the sources of clean water production and sanitation to promote sustainable economic development globally for the wellbeing of both all the people and nature. The importance of providing quality water cannot be over-emphasized, this is because access to clean drinking water and adequate discharge of waste water is vital for societal wellbeing and human existence, and access to clean and safe water is a fundamental human right to fulfill the requirements of the wellbeing of all humanity. The progress from MDGs to SDGs should be successful by the progress in achieving measurable outcome by underscoring the value of producing clean drinking water and sanitation to universalize human rights and human life in the planet earth. A new wave of innovation with new values to create safe renewable energy, quality water and a fully sanitized living environment has to be promoted as the bottom line for all humanity to come together with green and sustainable ecosystem full of hope and equal opportunities for all.

Acknowledgements

We would like to thank the DST/NRF SARChI (Innovation and Development) at the Tshwane University of Technology, Pretoria, South Africa for initiating the Science, Technology, Innovation Studies series of books in collaboration with African World Press.

We recognize and appreciate the support given by Dr. Jideofor Adibe, Adonis & Abbey Publishers Ltd, London, United Kingdom, which enabled publication of this book.

We also would like to thank the African Journal of Science, Technology, Innovation and Development (AJSTID) and extend our fullest appreciation and thanks to all the contributing authors.

Our sincere thanks to Ananthy Baskaran, the cover designer, and Jan B. Mwesigwa (www.janmwesigwa.com) our initial layout artist for their hard work and dedication to the book project.

Finally, we express our deepest appreciation and gratitude to Mr. Kassahun Checole and Mr. Girma A. Demeke, Africa World Press, Inc. & The Red Sea Press, Inc. for their cooperation and support during the publication process. We also thank all the publications staff at Africa World Press, Inc. & The Red Sea Press, Inc.

The DST/NRF Research Chair at Tshwane University of Technology and Africa World Press will promote the science, technology, innovation studies book series applying the principle to promote innovation and knowledge on and for Africa.

Chapter 1

Introduction

"Solutions to Access Safe and Drinking Water in Africa":

From MDGs to SDGs to Achieve Universal Access to Clean Water

Mammo Muchie & Angathevar Baskaran

The failure to provide food, shelter and safe drinking water with the provision of basic sanitation to all the people living in any part of this planet remains a big challenge to this day. This development failure has to change to bring development success in this century. Water is central for promoting social, economic and nature well being, development and transformation. Health, food, job creation, economic development and environmental protection depend on safe water and sanitation. It is remarkable that both the World Bank and the UN claim that 663 million people still do not have access to water sources that can provide safe and sanitised drinking water. The UN report claims that half of the population are in sub-Saharan Africa and about one-fifth live in South Asia.

The UN, WHO and UNICEF report that 780 million people do

not have access to clean drinking water. They claim that some 2.5 billion people lack access to sanitation protection and safety. They also report that, 2–5 million of the worlds's population especially children are exposed to death as a consequence of water related diseases annually. They die from preventable water related diseases every year (UN 2009; WHO and UNICEF, 2012). There have been efforts to explore and develop helpful explanations on a variety of issues such as water scarcity related to calculating how water demand exceeds the useable water supply, and the adequacy of the infrastructure to make water supply reliable. Something like 20% of the world's population (about 1.2 billion) is said to experience water scarcity (International Water Management Institute(IWMI), 2007)

The UN had set the Millenium Development Goals (MDGs) to halve the proportion of the population without improved drinking water between 1990 and 2015. The real question is whether the goal has been met in 2015 as expected, recognising that water is critical to realise the risk of failure by promoting a future where the basic necessities for human and nature wellbeing will be secure and sustainable. Today 91 per cent of the world's population is said to have access to better drinking water sources than before. This is 15 % more than what it was in 1990. The claim is that 2.6 billion people have access to piped drinking water making 58 % of the global population having such access to water on pipe. The UN reported that 147 countries from all parts of the world have reached the targets set by the MDGs.The only region that seems to have not met the targets is from Africa. The UN report says that Africa South of the Sahara met only 20 % of the proportion in gaining access to safe drinking water. Globally urban areas have 96 % and rural areas 84 % of the population to improved water resource access.

In the UN report the MDG goal on sanitation has not been as successful as access to safe drinking water sources. The number of those who live without access to better sanitation condition is reported to be as high as 2.4 billion people globally but with 70 % of those in Africa and 53 % of those in South Asia lacking access to improved sanitation. Despite the reported large number of people without access, the percentage with improved sanitation access globally is 68%. It is clear that most of the people without access to improved sanitation and hence not meeting the MDG targets are mainly in the developing world particularly in Africa and South Asia.

Sanitation and access to drinking safe water are intererlinked. When there is improved sanitation, gain to access to drinking safe and quality water will be open and available. Both the sources for clean water and managing human waste to avoid infecting the sources for the provision of sustainable clean and safe drinking water have to be dealt with equal measure.

The SDGs have now occupied the post-MDGs with goal 6 of the 17 goals combining access to clean water provision with sanitation. Goal 6 calls for the: "availability and sustainable management of water and sanitation for all" by including indicators and targets to remove open defecation for sanitation and the provision of better water quality. The expectation is that as the whole world has joined together there will be a global effort to create the condition for complete sanitation and water quality for the safety of the people of the world particularly in the areas of the world that performed not as well as those in the developed world. SDGs make water and sanitation as human rights providing universal and equitable access to safe, adequate, sustainable and affordable drinking water and essential sanitation and hygiene. That means to fail to have the right to drink water is a violation of human rights which means before and around 2030 all humans should have access to clean water and sanitation.

Every development challenge requires knowing how to create sustainable sanitation to protect, preserve, keep healthy, safe and manage the global water resources in order to maintain food security and the global phenomenon of rapidly growing urbanisation, the current risk of climate change, the provision of sustainable energy resources and promote the innovative wave of green economic development of hope. All in the world should collaborate to make sure all humanity have access to both clean quality water and sanitation. What was not achieved with the MDGs ought to be met fully before the SDGs target of 2030.

In this book a number of researchers have contributed towards this objective through their research. They discuss following specific areas of water and sanitation in Africa:

- Inequality in access to improved water and sanitation in Africa

- Treatment of abattoir wastewater using septic and multimedia anaerobic filtration tanks from a slaughter house
- Community view of public water projects and the challenges posed to state institutions
- Integrated Water Resources Management (IWRM) and challenges of microbiology quality of water resources
- Green drop certification of wastewater treatment plants to reduce drinking water sources pollution and bedrock of wastewater reuse
- Impact of climate change on water resources in Africa
- Treatment of the wastewater containing phenol and strontium using isolated cultures from mine water
- Technical challenges for water borehole design, construction and maintenance
- Political imperatives on water and wellbeing
- Impact of distance between on-site sanitation and location of boreholes on groundwater contamination
- Policy implication on water service indicators and basic household water service delivery in rural areas.

Oluwakemi S. Babatunde, Mammo Muchie & Angathevar Baskaran analyse the "Inequality in access to improved water and sanitation in Africa". They argue that access to sustainable water supply is tantamount to the aggregate wellbeing of individuals and states and therefore it is essential to understand the inequalities pervading Africans access to improved water and sanitation. They highlight that individuals and groups in Africa are denied reasonable access to water and basic sanitation, which replicates the discriminatory and marginalizing structure of the society. This discrimination can be on the bases of ethnicity, language, religion, gender, age, disability, differential water scheme, political injustice among many others.

Sometimes, the barrier preventing certain individuals and groups from having access to water and sanitation may be several discriminations, or the manifold impacts of various patterns of discrimination. For instance, an individual or group of a particular ethnic affiliation may lack access to water because of poverty and isolation (as a minor or a minority ethnic group). This can also be direct or indirect effects of discriminatory governmental laws and policies. This chapter therefore aims at discussing some of the inequalities prevalent in African societies with respect to access to improved water and sanitation.

Olanrewaju and Adewumi present findings from their research on the "treatment of abattoir wastewater using septic and multimedia anaerobic filtration tanks from a slaughter house in Akure, South-West Nigeria", by highlighting the potentiality of combining a septic and multi-media anaerobic filtration tanks to provide an efficient and economical treatment. In this chapter the feasibility study on the combination of physical, biological and chemical treatment processes using a wedge-wire screen, a two compartment septic tank and a multi-media anaerobic filtration tank with the addition of granulated activated carbon as an absorption media in the filtration tank was investigated. The study was based on economic analysis of the capital cost (design, purchase and installation costs) and running costs (operation and maintenance) of abattoir wastewater treatment plant, costs and benefits of the treatment unit. The authors revealed and recommended that the proposed technology has good potential to reduce substantially the pollution load of slaughter house effluents.

Akpabio examines findings on "community view of public water projects and the challenges posed to state institutions in Nigeria". The chapter was aimed at investigating how cultural issues contend with formal State initiatives for efficient water resources management in Akwa Ibom State, Nigeria. The study used key contending State water management principles, (water rights, cost recovery and environmental sustainability) to compare with local practice to observe where there are commonalities and differences. The study highlights the fact that since there is relative abundance of water in the study area, which may not elicit fullest interest on government projects from the communities examined, a more rational approach to handle such situations by government agencies should be based on demand responsive project targeting approach. Although, the influence of ecological factors dictated the citing of projects in the study areas, the study revealed that such assumption is not fruitful where traditional attitudes predominate, in addition to the non-appreciation of the 'scarcity value' of water by the affected communities.

Adeleke and Bezuidenhout explored "integrated water resources management (IWRM) in South Africa: challenges of microbiology quality of water resources". The report looked at the framework of IWRM in South Africa and microbiological quality of South African water resources. The authors also discussed, other programmes, such as the National Microbial Water Quality Programme (NMMP), and the green and blue drop certifications. The chapter highlights the major elements of the South African water policy and how IWRM is currently managed. It mentioned problems such as, inability of water managers to properly translate the written forms of IWRM concepts into practical forms, institutional challenges that persist as a result of insufficient alignment and cooperation between the policies of different government departments and the practices of different water sectors that impact on water as some of the challenges facing IWRM in South Africa. In addition the authors reported that having realised the enormous problems associated with the quality of South African water; the South African Department of Water Affairs introduced two different certification programmes; the Blue drop and the Green drop, which were initiated in 2005 and 2008, respectively.

Furthermore, the study on "South African Green Drop Evaluation and its possible implication in water supply of the country via wastewater reuse" by Adewumi and Olanrewaju presents the results of the first assessment of wastewater treatment plants in South Africa and the implication on wastewater reuse in water scarce areas of the country. The findings revealed that many of the wastewater treatment works failed to meet the requirements for the award of Green Drop Certificate. This was reported to be due to poor management style and ageing infrastructure. According to the evaluation equation, the lowest cumulative risk rating (CRR) that can be achieved is 1 (No risks) and the highest is 48 (Very high risky). The First Order Assessment indicated that none of the WWTWs assessed approached the highest possible risk value of 48. Despite the observed high risks ratings (CRR of 18–28), none of the WWTWs was in the state of total collapse. The authors proposed that adequate maintenance to meet the set criteria will reduce drinking water source pollution and provide a solid foundation for alternative source of water for non potable purposes through reuse.

Akpor and Boakye on the "impact of climate change on Africa water resources", current impacts of climate change on Africa water resources, vulnerability and current climate change adaptation steps in Africa were discussed. It also reports that historically, Africa climate change record shows an approximate 0.7°C warming over most of the twelfth century, with a decrease in rainfall over large parts of the Sahel and an increase in rainfall in East Central Africa. The authors further argued that despite the fact that no conclusive evidence was yet to be available to substantiate the cause and effect relationship of climate change and water resources, given the current African vulnerability level and its effects on the economy and food security, it is obvious that the negative impacts will be greatest in Africa. In conclusion, the chapter asserts that the effects of climate change, such as changes in floods and drought patterns, poor water quality and decrease in surface and ground water are real, with impacts already affecting people, ecosystems and biodiversities in Africa.

Oborien analyses the "treatment of wastewater containing phenol and strontium using isolated cultures from mine water" and shows that wastewater containing organic radioactive compounds is produced by the nuclear, medical, industrial, agricultural, and food processing industries, either as part of the product or as a byproduct of the manufacturing process, hence release of radioactive wastes from the above mentioned activities still poses many problems to human life and the natural environment. The study investigated phenol degradation capability of microbial isolate cultures under radionuclide exposure conditions in batch systems using simple media. The study reports that the isolated cultures were able to degrade phenol in the presence of strontium in the simulated organic radioactive waste. The study also reports that phenol biodegradation in the entire range of initial phenol concentration that was investigated in during the study.

Nwankwoala and Udom discuss the "Technical challenges for water borehole design, construction and maintenance in the Eastern Niger Delta of Nigeria". They highlight the fact that in the Eastern Niger Delta region of Nigeria, boreholes are drilled haphazardly and without coordination leading to numerous cases of abandoned wells. This un wellcome trend results from lack of technical inputs into the design, materials and effective supervision, as well as general lack of geologic and hydrogeologic knowledge of the area, resulting in high rate of borehole failure as well as poor performance and yield. They argue that the geological and hydrogeological challenges, coupled with the difficult environmental terrain required highly experienced professionals. Therefore they highlight the hydrogeologic uncertainties as well as technical realities for sustainable water supply borehole construction and maintenance. They also suggest sustainable options for borehole design, drilling, completion and development in the Eastern Niger Delta region.

Oshewolo, Muchie and Baskaran provide some "Reflections on water and wellbeing: the political imperatives in Nigeria". They draw attention to the fact that African countries have consistently been ranked as countries with the least sustainable access to improved water sources such as piped water into dwelling, yard or plot, public tap or standpipe, tubewell or borehole, protected spring, and hygienic collection of rain water. Then they analyse the worsening situation in Nigeria, where the current water supply service coverage in the country is only 58 per cent, and women and children have to trek long distances to fetch water from streams and ponds which are most times contaminated. They highlight that the situation is more frightening in the rural areas with only 42 per cent having access to potable water supply in the rural areas. To address this challenge, this chapter argues that the huge financing gap in the water sector must be effectively bridged. Aside from funding, other issues begging for policy attention include the moral commitment of the political actors to the realization of sectoral policy guidelines, water sector planning, data generation, monitoring and evaluation, accountability and the strengthening of institutional mechanism.

Matodzi M Mokoena & Murembiwa S. Mukhola discuss the "Impact of distance between on-site sanitation and location of boreholes on groundwater contamination: the case of developing and semi-developed rural areas of Limpopo Province, South Africa." It analyses the impact of on-site sanitation and animal droppings on the faecal pollution of the boreholes in the yards. Contamination of the groundwater by E. coli was found to be higher at a distance of less than 20 m away from a pit latrine than at a distance of up to 30 m away; for Enterococci it was found that there was less contamination at a distance of less than 20 m than that of between >20 m and <30 m. They found that pit latrines and animal droppings randomly distributed in the yard contribute to contaminating the water of the boreholes. They concluder that yard planning is needed when building new houses, pit latrines should be situated at least 30 m away from boreholes, and animals should not be kept within reach of boreholes.

Finally, Mudau, Mukhola and Hunter provide "analysis of policy implication on water service indicators and basic household water service delivery in rural areas of South Africa". They found that despite the availability of indicators, rural communities still spend more time collecting water from the street. Apparently they travel beyond the limits to access safe water for domestic use. However the service rendered is composed of major disturbances that result in absence of water services for days; exposing them to health risks. Currently there is no methodology that is used by WSA's to measure the level of water service based on these indicators; in localized rural communities that depend on tap water accessed from the street. The authors propose an estimate measurement in which WSA's could quantify its performance on basic household water service delivery in rural areas of SA. They highlight that water which is accessible, available, potable, affordable and reliable is crucial to the service rendered to communities. Where sufficient water cannot be provided, waters safety plans at household level should be employed for public health gains.

Together the research contributions in this book highlight the importance of water as an essential natural source, hence the need for effective management, both in terms of quality and quantity, since reduction in the availability of water can lead to adverse health, environmental and social effects, hence the need to conserve water, pollute less, manage supply and demand, and slow population growth. These principles reflect the importance of water in our daily lives and the need for proper communication, gender equity, and economic and policy incentives to manage the resource properly. In conclusion, the contributors illustrate the need to realise the fact that water-related challenges cannot be solved by quick technical solutions, but through the consideration of cultural, educational, communication and scientific aspects.

References

International Water Management Institute (2007), *Water for Food, Water for Life: A Comprehensive Assessment of Water Management in Agriculture*. London: Earthscan.

Molden, D. (ed.) (2007), *A Comprehensive Assessment of Water Management in Agriculture*, Sterling, VA, and London: International Water Management Institute. Available at: http://www.fao.org/nr/water/docs/summary_synthesisbook.pdf

UNICEF and World Health Organization (2012), *Progress on Drinking Water and Sanitation*. Available at: https://www.unicef.org/media/files/JMPreport2012.pdf

United Nations (2009), *World Water Development Report (WWDR3): Water in a Changing World*. Available at: http://www.unwater.org/publications/publications-detail/ en/c/202716/

Chapter 2

Inequality in Access to Improved Water and Sanitation in Africa

Oluwakemi S. Babatunde, Angathevar Baskaran & Mammo Muchie

1. Introduction

In Africa, as in many countries of the world, inequality is the norm of basic social existence. Inequality is a universal social phenomenon that denotes the existence of actual or illusory struggle for 'scarce' social goods which are unevenly distributed among members of a society. Although water is commonly seen as naturally given and abundant, water, in its clean state, is one of the rarest elements in the world (Omole and Longe, 2008). It is a scarce societal resource in as much as it is not equally available to individuals in society. It is estimated that a meager of three percent of the world's total water is fresh, 2.5 percent of which is frozen, unavailable and inaccessible by man (World Business Council for Sustainable Development, (WBCSD) 2006). Wherever it is available, it is inequitably accessible by individuals when and where they need it; Water is also managed according to varied established social laws.

Non-availability of water though an apparent natural problem is yet compounded by social, demographic, political and economic factors. These are reflected in growing populations and urbanization; higher standards of living and the relative increase in the demand for water; structural problems and competition for available freshwater between the various sectors in the society such as households, industries, municipals, agriculture and even between nations that share watercourses (Falkenmark et al., 1989). Access to sustainable water supply is tantamount to the aggregate wellbeing of individuals and states. Therefore it is essential to understand the inequalities pervading Africans access to improved water and sanitation.

According to the Global Water Supply and Sanitation Assessment, a reasonable access to water implies that an individual is at ease of using at least twenty liters of water per day from a source within one kilometer of his/her home, while basic sanitation denotes private or shared but not public disposal systems that separate waste from human contact (GWSSAR, 2000). However, individuals and groups in Africa are denied reasonable access to water and basic sanitation. This to some extent replicate the discriminatory and marginalizing structure of the society. This discrimination can be on the bases of ethnicity, language, religion, gender, age, disability, differential water scheme, political injustice among many others. Sometimes, the barrier preventing certain individuals and groups from having access to water and sanitation may be several discriminations, or the manifold impacts of various patterns of discrimination. For instance, an individual or group of a particular ethnic affiliation may lack access to water because of poverty and isolation (as a minor or a minority ethnic group). This can also be direct or indirect effects of discriminatory governmental laws and policies. This chapter was therefore aimed at discussing some of the inequalities prevalent in African societies with respect to access to improved water and sanitation.

2. Geographical Inequality

Despite the varieties of water resources (springs, rivers, lakes) in Africa, it is deemed the second driest in the globe. Freshwater is unequally distributed across countries and regions and a large number of Africa's rivers and lake basins are also shared by two or more countries. The continents renewable water resources represent a meager estimate of nine percent (3,931 km^3) of the world's total freshwater resources. In 2008, the continental annual average water availability per person was 4 008 m^3, below the global average of 6,498 m^3 per capita. This is due in large part to climatic erraticism which is made worse by series of floods, droughts and the surge in human population (Food and Agriculture Organization (FAO), 2009). Table 1 shows the disparities in the availability of fresh water resources across some regions of the globe.

Table 1: Geographical Distribution of Internal Renewable Freshwater Resources by World Regions

Continent/ Region	Volume per Year (km^3 10^{9}m^3)	Percentage of World Freshwater Resources	Per Capita (m^3/year) 2008
World	43 802	100.0	6 498
Africa	3 931	9.0	4 008
Asia	12 393	28.3	3 037
South America	12 380	28.3	32 165
Central America and Caribbean	781	1.8	9 645
North America	6 877	15.7	15 166
Oceania	892	2.0	32 366
Europe	6 548	14.9	8 941

Source: Adapted and modified from United Nations Environment Programme (UNEP), 2010.

As shown in Table 1, Asia and South America has most of the fresh water available in the world with 28.3 percent, followed by North America and Europe at 15.7% and 14.9% respectively. Though the percentage of water availability in Africa (9%) is higher than in the Caribbean (2%) and Oceania (1.8%), it is not enough for its giant population

Although water scarcity threatens all of African countries, different nation states and regions face different constraints and opportunities. Africa's groundwater resources represent only 15 per cent of total renewable water resources; yet, these supply approximately 75 percent of its population with most of its drinking water. Consequently, many have resorted to other surface sources (rivers, lakes, dams, streams, ponds) and in so doing, experience the problems that accompany treating such water (United Nations Environment Programme (UNEP), 2010). Table 2 shows the comparative renewable water resources in Africa's sub-regions.

Table 2: Geographical Distribution of Renewable Freshwater Resources in Africa

Africa's Sub Region	Total water Resource (km^3/year) (2008)	Percentage of Internal water Resources of Africa
Central Africa	2858.08	50.66
Eastern Africa	262.04	4.64
Western, Indian Ocean Islands	345.95	6.13
Northern Africa	168.66	2.99
Southern Africa	691.35	12.25
Western Africa	1 315.28	23.32
Total	5 641.36	100

Source: Adapted and modified from United Nations Environment Programme (UNEP), 2010.

African countries with the least access to water resources are in the Northern, Southern and Eastern Africa while Central and Western African countries have the most access to water. Though the latter have adequate surface and ground water resources to meet most of the countries' demands for potable water, these are unequally distributed leading to scarcity in some regions and locations. In the northern towns of Nigeria as in other arid African regions, water resources have become so depleted and/or contaminated that they are unable to meet increasing demands.

3. Inequality in Water Distribution

Water is not evenly distributed across the globe as an estimated 20 percent of the world's population lack access to safe drinking water

(Simonovic, 2000), and 50 percent of the world's population lack access to sanitation (Cosgrove and Rijsberman, 2000). In all regions of Africa (except central Africa), water availability per person is below global averages. In 2006, it was estimated that 341 million people in Africa lacked access to improved drinking water sources (WHO/UNICEF, 2008). In 2010, 60 percent of African population lacked access to improved sanitation facilities, while 34 percent had no access to improved drinking water sources. In sub-Saharan Africa, 69 percent of the population has no proper sanitation facilities, while 40 percent has no reliable improved water source (WHO/UNICEF, 2012).

Only users of 'improved' drinking water sources are considered having 'access to drinking water'. Improved drinking water sources are defined as those by nature of their construction or through active intervention are protected from outside contamination, particularly from contamination with fecal matter (WHO/UNICEF, 2008), while the unimproved water sources are opened and unprotected from contaminations. Examples of improved water sources include; Piped water located inside the user's the dwelling, plot or yard, public taps or standpipes, boreholes or tube wells, protected dug wells, protected springs, and rainwater (WHO/UNICEF, 2011). Also, individuals who use 'improved' sanitation facilities only are considered to have 'access to sanitation'. Improved sanitation facility denotes one that hygienically separates human excreta from human contact. They include: Flush or Pour-flush that empties into a) Piped sewer system, b) Septic tank, c) Pit latrine; Ventilated Improved Pit latrine (VIP); Pit latrine with slab and Composting toilet.

Africa water and sanitation problems are severe due to increasing population, massive urbanization with improper planning, industrial development, and improved standard of living as said earlier. Perverse inequalities in access to water and sanitation exist between the urban and rural populations. Usually, the drinking water situation and sanitations are worse in rural areas than in urban ones. This however accentuates the global awareness that rural populations persistently have lower levels of access than urban populations. The average urban drinking water coverage in Africa is 85 per cent while only 51 percent of people in rural areas have access to improved drinking water though it has a higher per cent of its population in rural areas (WHO/UNICEF, 2008 cited in UNEP, 2010). As at 2010, 85 per cent of population in urban areas had access to improved water sources with 54 per cent in the rural areas. Access to improved sanitation also showed this disparity as record showed that 54 per cent of urban settlers used improved sanitation while 31 per cent of rural dwellers did not (WHO/UNICEF, 2012). The percentage distribution of urban and rural population with improved sources of drinking water and sanitation is shown in Figure 1.

Figure 1: Progress on Drinking Water and Sanitation (A: population with access to improved drinking, B: population with access to improved sanitation)

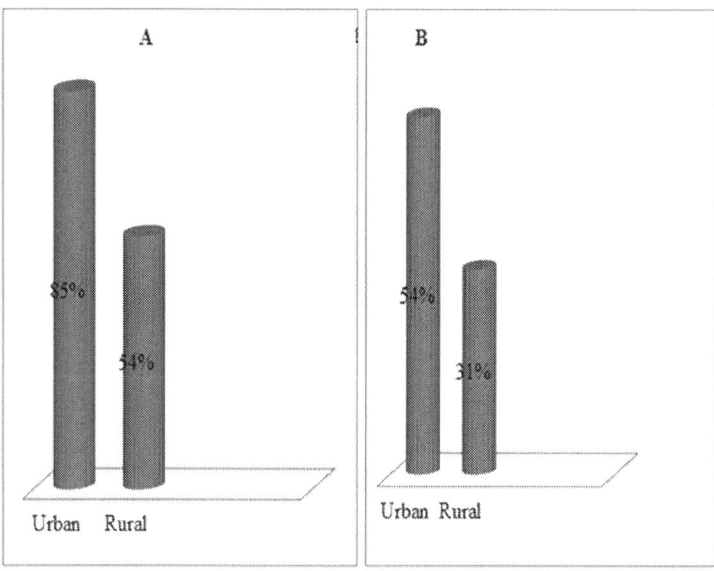

Source: Adapted and modified from WHO/UNICEF, 2012.

These rural areas are often the geographically removed, remote and marginalized regions, habitually ignored in planning. This perpetuates the horror of poverty and underdevelopment in most rural regions of Africa. Also, slum dwellers frequently lack access to adequate water and sanitation due to their deliberate exclusion from formal water services in most countries' laws and policies.

4. Wealth Inequality and Access to Water and Sanitation

Access to improved water and sanitation in Africa and especially sub-Saharan Africa is highly correlated with wealth and the effects of this are often different due to variations in peoples' experiences of poverty. Poverty is widespread in Africa: daily, nearly half of the entire population of Africa lives on less than one dollar per person (African Development Bank (AfDB), 2009). Dimensions of poverty include among others; income and consumption, health, sustainable livelihood, security and vulnerability, inclusion and empowerment (Hirji et al., 2002).

Whereas poverty is a causative factor in the pervasive lack of access to improved water sources and sanitation; wealth is often tied to the overconsumption of water resources. A poor family of eight living in a squatter camp in the Cape Town area of South Africa was said to use about 120 liters of water per day while, a couple living in a rich neighbourhood with a big garden to water, could use 2000 liters per day (Pallett, 1997). Socioeconomic status of a group is obtained by dividing the population into five equal parts/quintiles (from the poorest to the richest) using the wealth index/asset index which is made up of different assets, comprising among other things; type of dwelling, roofing materials, flooring type, hectares of land, means of transportation, number of animals, television, refrigerator and radio. It has been estimated that the richest quintile of the population in sub-Saharan Africa is more than twice likely as the poorest quintile to use an improved drinking water source. The comforts and benefits of piped water on premises are also solely enjoyed by the wealthiest. This is further demonstrated in Figure 2

Figure 2: Drinking water coverage by wealth quintiles in sub-Saharan Africa

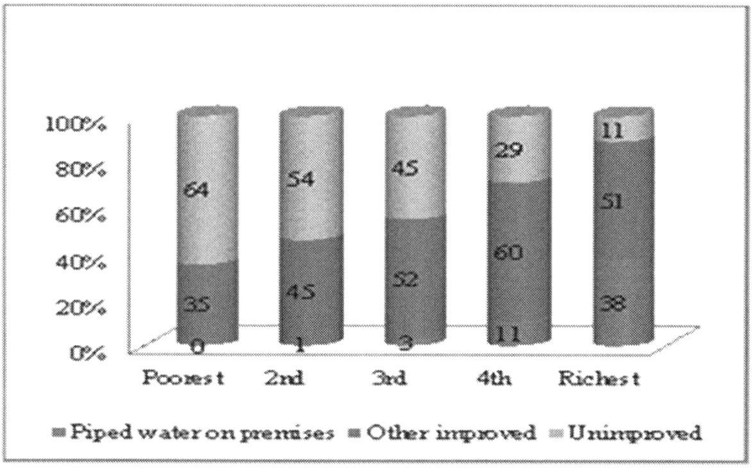

Source: Adapted and modified from MICS and DHS surveys from 35 countries in sub-Saharan Africa, 2004-2009, in WHO/UNICEF, 2012.

Additionally, the richest quintile is estimated to be five times more likely to use an improved sanitation facility than the poorest quintile while the latter is around sixteen times as likely to practice open defecation as the richest quintile. Nonetheless, three percent of the richest quintile practices open defecation (WHO/UNICEF, 2010). This is further illustrated in Figure 3.

It's been estimated also that persons in rural areas in sub-Saharan Africa spend more than thirty minutes on single water collection trip than those in urban areas while the urban poor spend greater time collecting water than their richer neighbours who are three times more likely to have a piped supply in place. Also, people in poor densely populated areas (usually the poor) expend long periods of time queuing at public taps, boreholes and wells to fetch water.

Figure 3: Sanitation by wealth quintiles in sub-Saharan Africa

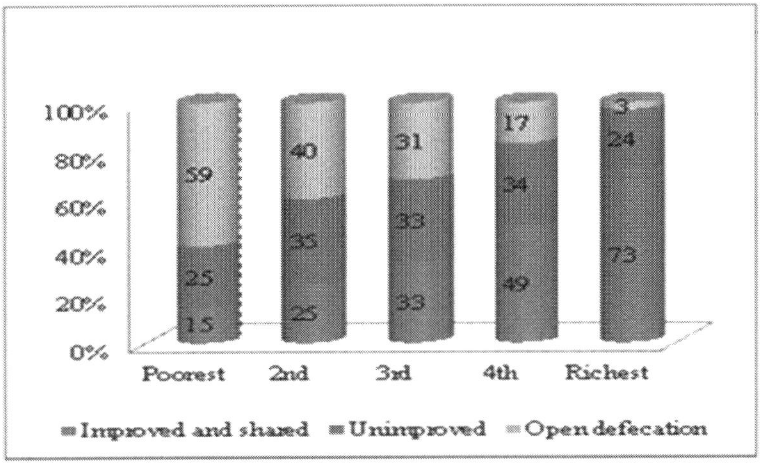

Source: Adapted and modified from MICS and DHS surveys from 35 countries in sub-Saharan Africa, 2004-2009, in WHO/UNICEF, 2012.

5. Gender Inequality and Access to Water

Africa is ridden with discrimination based on sex/gender and age; evidence shows that women and girls in all strata of society face mammoth barriers and risks in accessing water. By tradition, women and young children, especially girls, are instrumental in providing water for their families, particularly in rural Africa which limits their time for other productive activities, including education, work and rest. They approximately perform between 65 and 72 per cent of water collection duties (WHO/UNICEF, 2008). They are thus more adversely affected when there is limited access to water resources spending as much as 40 percent of their daily nutritional intake travelling to collect water (Chenje, 2000). They often fetch and carry water in containers from long distances, spending large amounts of time and energy. A graphic illustration of water collection responsibilities is shown in Figure 4.

By tradition in many rural societies also, women and girls are often required to stay away from using shared sanitation facilities except during dark hours while some are not even allowed to use these facilities at all. This forces some women and girls to travel long distance out of the peering eyes of the men to fulfill their sanitation needs. This endangers their personal safety, reduces their dignity and hampers their health. Teenage girls also need easy access to safe water, toilets and washrooms. This is to enable them maintain privacy and manage menstruation which will invariably boost their self-worth. However, these are often lacking in most rural schools. Little wonder then why girls skip schools during menstruation and drop out eventually as a result of poor performance. Women and girls are indoctrinated into believing they should see themselves less than their male counterparts in a bid to show their submissiveness and caring nature, thus most of them willingly deny themselves the use of safe water and sanitation in order to satisfy the males who are believed superior.

Figure 4: Water Collection Responsibilities by Gender in Africa

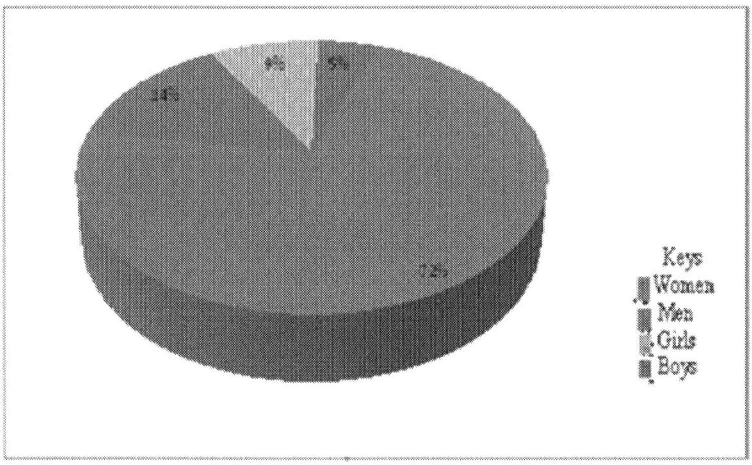

Source: Adapted and modified from WHO/UNICEF 2008: Progress on Drinking Water and Sanitation Special focus on Sanitation. Joint Monitoring Programme, (JMP).

6. Water Policies, Institutional and Legal Frameworks in Africa

'The world water crisis is a crisis of governance...there is enough water to provide water security for all, but only if we change the way we manage and develop it' (HRH the Prince of Orange 2002). All African countries in collaboration with international agencies are currently increasing their political and financial commitments and efforts toward ensuring that Africans have more access to safe water and sanitation. However, these efforts are usually inadequate especially in sub-Saharan Africa as the different policy measures and institutional arrangements seldom sustain viable management of water resources.

Most African countries do not see access to safe water and sanitation as a fundamental right of individuals, as a result it is not explicitly written in their constitutions. Though water policy is the basis for legislation, strategic planning and operational management of water resources, it is saddening that some African countries do not have national water policies, while many that have are recently adopted. In most countries where these policies exist, they are often inadequate, leading to poor water management.

Significant steps toward effective management of water resources started with the creation of the National Water Resources Institute (NWRI), the River Basin Development Authorities (RBDA) in 1976 and the Federal Ministry of Water Resources (FMWR) in 1977. While FMWR was responsible for formulating policy and advising, the NWRI was set up primarily for research, to promote the establishment of a uniform national data collection system relating to surface and subsurface water resources and manpower training. These, it is yet to fulfill due to reasons including; lack of funds, shortage of skilled manpower, and inadequate equipment among others. The RBDAs were responsible for the provision of water to communities for agricultural, domestic, and industrial use in their basin areas (FMWR, 2007). The RBDAs are backed up by the RBDA act of 1986 and a subsidiary of the FMWR (Kuruk, 2005).

The 1989 National Policy on Environment related water resources management to catchment basins as the basic unit of analysis in water management. These basins were managed by RBDAs which are parastatals under the Federal Ministry of Agriculture and Water Resources (FMAWR). The FMAWR is with the general responsibility of managing the country's water resources by promoting the optimum planning, development and use of Nigeria's water resources and by ensuring the coordination of all activities that are expected to influence the quality, quantity, distribution, use and management of water resources. In addition, the ministry is tasked for ensuring the application of appropriate standards and techniques for the investigation, utilization, control, protection, management and administration of water resources. The Federal Environmental Protection Agency, (FEPA) was established in 1988, and became the Federal Ministry of Environment in 1999 (Adelegan, 2004).

The management of water resources at this time was largely rife with problems some of which are prevalent today. They are: shortage of water; needless duplication and overlap in organizations, structures and functions of the relevant water bodies; ill-defined and uncoordinated roles of the Federal, State and Local Government agencies responsible for water resources development; failure to recognize the inter-relationship between surface and ground waters, between water resources and land use and lack of effective water and environmental protection laws, and the means to enforce the already existing laws (FGN, 1988).

One of the most effective water regulations in Nigeria today is the Water Resources Decree of 1993 (FGN, 1993). Though it acknowledged customary laws relating to water rights, it nevertheless stated that water is owned by the nation, managed and controlled by the Federal Ministry of Water Resources (FMWR, 2003). Section 1(i) of the Water resources decree vests in the Federal Government the right to the use and control of all surface and groundwater and all water in any water-course that involve more than a state, for the purpose of promoting the planning, development and use of the country's water resources; coordinating the distribution, use and management of water resources; and ensuring the application of appropriate standards for the investigation, use, control, protection of water resources.

Section 2 of the Water Resources Decree, states that any person may:

i. take water without charge for his domestic purpose or for watering his livestock from any water course to which the public has free access; or

ii. may use water for the purpose of fishing or for navigation to the extent that such use is not inconsistent with any other law for the time being in force; or

iii. who, has a statutory or customary right of occupancy to any land, may take and use water from the underground water source or if adjoining on the bank of any water course, from that watercourse, without charge for domestic purposes, for watering livestock and for personal irrigation schemes (FGN, 1993).

As defined in the Water Resources decree, the term "domestic use" implies the use of water for drinking, cooking, washing, bathing, cooling, gardening, or for any other domestic purpose in any residential premises utilized for non-profit motives, "non-domestic use" denotes the use of water from any waterworks for profit or gain.; while the term "public use" refers to any domestic or agricultural use from any waterworks provided through any fountain, standpipe, valve, tap or appliance used. The decree, failed to recognize the fact that the irrational exploitation of underground water resources with no recourse to expert evaluation could lead to other adverse environmental occurrences, like subsidence and landslides, among other things, if overexploited (Oteri and Atolagbe, 2003).

Section 9 (1) of the decree also stipulated that the diversion, storage, pumping or use on a commercial scale of any water or the construction, maintenance, operation, repair of any bore-hole or any hydraulic works shall be carried out only in accordance with a license issued pursuant to the regulations made under the decree. It went further in subsection (2) in stating that a "person in breach of the provisions of subsection (1) of this section commits an offence under this Decree". Obviously now in Nigeria, particularly in peri-urban and rural areas, people indiscriminately dig wells without any or much sanction and without informed directives.

The decree put all power over water resources within an area covered by the certificate of occupancy (with the exception of interstate water courses) on any individual who can secure it either through the government or customary means. Authority on landed matters and land ownership in Nigeria is fraught with problems. These problems arise from the overriding authority of the Federal authority backed up by the Land Use Act of 1978 and the less influential traditional/historical authority of the ownership of land by individuals, backed up by customary laws. The Act vests "all land comprised in the territory of each State (except land vested in the Federal Government or its agencies) solely in the Governor of the State, who would hold such land in trust for the people" Land Use Act (1978). The Local Government can also grant customary rights of occupancy on land not situated in urban areas, to any person or organization for the use of land in the Local Government Area (Kuruk, 2005). Though customary (traditional) rights to land ownership are instituted in customary laws and backed up by Federal laws, they are subjected to them.

The Water Resource Decree is also not gritty enough in ensuring that water is kept safe and that violators are severely dealt with. The punitive measures contained in Section 18 of the decree are too palliative and they won't serve as any deterrent to would be offenders. Subsection (1) and (2) states "any person who contravenes or fails to comply with any provisions of this Decree, or any regulation, made thereunder commits an offence and is liable upon conviction to a fine not exceeding 2,000 naira or to a term of imprisonment not exceeding six months or to both such fine and imprisonment, and, in the case of a continuing offence to an additional fine not exceeding 100 naira for every day or part of a day that the offence continues"; "where an offence under this Decree has been committed by a body corporate or firm or other association of individuals, a person who at the time of the commission of the offence was any officer thereof or was purporting to act in such capacity is severally guilty of that offence and liable to be prosecuted against and punished for the offence in like manner as if he had himself committed the offence, unless he proves that the act or omission constituting the offence took place without his knowledge, consent or connivance" (FGN, 1993). The costs of treating water do not commensurate the penalties stated above, little wonder then that industries, groups and individuals gallantly flaunt water regulations. This also shows that most of the laws on water pollution, standards and regulations are façade with not genuine intent in preserving and sustaining the environment.

As in many African countries, statutory water laws in Nigeria conflict with the customary laws just as it is the case with land ownership. The exclusive legislative powers and the concurrent responsibilities for water resources of the three tiers of government, Federal, State and Local also breeds divisions and contribute to the lack of inter-sectoral organization with all sectors pursuing independent water agendas, engendering problems to coordination and description of roles. The Federal, State and Local government are saddled with the responsibilities of formulating and coordinating national water policies, development and management of large water resources infrastructure, dams reservoirs, irrigation and water supply schemes; providing potable water supply (through State Water Agencies (SWAs) and providing rural water supplies and sanitation facilities respectively to individuals and groups in Nigeria.

The National Water Supply and Sanitation Policy of 2000 focuses on the provision of sufficient potable water and adequate sanitation to all Nigerians in an affordable and sustainable way through participatory investment by the three tiers of government, the private sector and the beneficiary; adequate supply of good quality, affordable water and sanitation services as a basic human need; privatization of water supply and wastewater services (where feasible) with adequate protection for the poor. Strategies highlighted to achieve these include among others: metering of all water supply schemes; recovery of economic rates with welfare service for the poor; protection of traditional water supply sources and promotion of traditional water quality practices; rural communities shall take full ownership of water supply facilities provided by the Government; private sector participation in the water supply industry; and water shall be managed at the lowest appropriate level (See NWSSP, 2000: item 17, 19, and 20).

This policy defined water as an economic good. The various government subsidies on water have often been justified on the ground of thoughtfulness of affordability by the poor. However, these have often proved ineffective in helping the poor, while the upper and middle classes benefit more from subsidized services as most of the poor have no access to improved water and sanitation facilities as the less poor.

7. Conclusion

Notwithstanding the concerted efforts of governments and international agencies in many African countries, improved water supply and sanitation coverage is still a mirage. Most national legal and institutional frameworks remain undeveloped. This is mainly due to too many incongruent policies and agencies that bear no responsibilities for sustainable improved water and sanitation delivery. Other reasons include: rate of socioeconomic development that far outweighs the level of water supply and sanitation, corruption, pitiable service delivery orientation, poor data collection and monitoring, epileptic power supply, poor maintenance and management culture which accounts for the regular breakdown of water and sanitation facilities.

There is need for African governments and all agencies to recommit themselves to the development of groundwater and surface resources. The tenacity with which laws and policies are formulated should be introduced into the management and monitoring of their implementations at all levels to ensure discipline and accountability financially and otherwise. Besides, water and sanitation services should be reliable and prices should aim at improving water resources management, sanitation and efficiency in the use of water and sanitation facilities. People should also be educated on the essence of safe water and sanitation and incentives provided to encourage voluntary water and environmental protection.

References

Adelegan, J.A. (2004), *The History of Environmental Policy and Pollution of Water Sources in Nigeria (1960-2004): The Way Forward*, Available at: http://web.fu-berlin.de/ffu/akumwelt/bc2004/download/adelegan_f.pdf (Accessed 8/11/2013).

AfDB (2009), 'Gender, Poverty and Environmental Indicators on African Countries', Economic and Social in Africa Water Atlas (Division of Early Warning and Assessment (DEWA), United Nations Environment Programme), Nairobi, Kenya.

Chenje, M. (2000), 'State of the Environment Zambezi Basin', Southern African Research & Documentation Centre, Zimbabwe in Africa Water Atlas (Division of Early Warning and Assessment (DEWA), United Nations Environment Programme), Nairobi, Kenya.

Cosgrove, J. and Rijsberman, F. (2000), *World Water Vision: Making Water Everybody's Business*, Earthscan, UK. Available at: http://www.watervision.org (Accessed 1/11/2013).

Falkenmark, M., Lundqvist, J. and Widstrand, C. (1989), 'Macro-scale water scarcity requires micro-scale approaches: Aspects of vulnerability in semi- arid development', in *Nat. Resource Forum*, 13: 258–267.

FAO (2009), 'AQUASTAT Database', Food and Agriculture Organization of the United Nations, Available at: http://www.fao.org/nr/aquastat (Accessed on 5/11/2013).

Federal Government of Nigeria (FGN) (1988), *Harmful Wastes Decree No. 42 of November 30, 1988,* Federal Government of Nigeria, Lagos: Government Press.

______ (1993), *Nigeria: Water Resources Decree 1993, Decree No.101*. Available at: www.ielrc.org/content/e9302.pdf (Accessed 9/11/2013).

FMWR (2003), 'Water Resources Management Institutions in Nigeria: Institutional Mapping Report', Draft Report, Abuja: FMRW.

______ (2007), 'Federal Ministry of Water Resources: Organization and Activities', Federal Republic of Nigeria. Available at: http://aochycos.ird.ne/html/partnat/fedwater/index.htm (Accessed 8/11/2013).

Global Water Supply and Sanitation Assessment Report (GWSSAR) (2000), In: World Business Council for Sustainable Development (WBCSD), 2006: Water Facts and Trends. Available at: http://www.wbcsd.org (Accessed 1/11/2013)

Hirji, R., Johnson, P., Maro, P. and Matiza-Chiuta, T. (2002), *Defining and Mainstreaming Environmental Sustainability in Water Resource Management in Southern Africa*, Washington, DC: World Bank.

HRH the Prince of Orange (2002), 'No Water No Future: A Water Focus for Johannesburg', Consultative Group on International Agriculture, Available at: http://www.cgiar.org/iwmi/accra2002/NoWaterNoFuture.pdf, (Accessed 8/11/2013)

Kuruk, P. (2005), *Customary Water Laws and Practices: Nigeria*, Available at: http://www.fao.org/Legal/advserv/FAOI-UCNcs/Nigeria.pdf. (Accessed 8/11/2013)

National Water Supply and Sanitation Policy (2000), Document of Federal Ministry of Water Resources, Abuja, Nigeria.

Omole, D.O. and Longe, E.O. (2008), 'An Assessment of the Impact of Abattoir Effluents on River Illo, Ota, Nigeria', in *Journal of Environmental Science and Technology,* 1(2): 56-54.

Oteri, A. and Atolagbe, F. (2003), 'Saltwater Intrusion into Coastal Aquifers in Nigeria', *The Second International Conference on Saltwater Intrusion and Coastal Aquifers-Monitoring, Modeling, and Management,* Mérida, Yucatán, México.

Pallett, J. (1997), *Sharing Water in Southern Africa*, Windhoek: Desert Research Foundation of Namibia.

Simonovic, S. P. (2000), 'Tools for Water Management: one view of the future', in *Water International*, 25: 76-88.

UNEP (2010), Africa *Water Atlas* (Division of Early Warning and Assessment (DEWA), United Nations Environment Programme), Nairobi, Kenya. Available at: 29/11/2011).

UNICEF/WHO (2011), 'Drinking Water Equity, Safety and Sustainability: Thematic Report on Drinking Water', Available at: http://www.wssinfo.org (Accessed 5/11/2013).

WHO/UNICEF (2008), 'Progress on Drinking Water and Sanitation, Special focus on Sanitation: Joint Monitoring Programme', Available at: http://www.wssinfo.org (Accessed 5/11/2013).

________ (2010), 'Multiple Indicator Cluster Surveys (MICS) and

Demographic and Health Surveys (DHS) from 33 countries in sub-Saharan Africa, 2004-2009', Joint Monitoring Programme for Water Supply and Sanitation.

________ (2012), 'Progress on Drinking Water and Sanitation, Special focus on Sanitation', Joint Monitoring Programme (JMP), Available at: http://www.who.int/water_sanitation_health (Accessed 5/11/2013).

World Business Council for Sustainable Development (WBCSD) (2006), Water Facts and Trends. Available at: http://www.wbcsd.org (Accessed 1/11/2013)

Chapter 3

Treatment of Abattoir Wastewater Using Septic and Multimedia Anaerobic Filtration Tanks from a Slaughter House in Akure, South-West Nigeria

Olawale O. Olanrewaju & James R. Adewumi

1. Introduction

In most cities of Nigeria, abattoirs are situated in residential areas because of the demand for fresh meat. However, most of these abattoirs lack functioning waste treatment facilities, hence they dispose their wastes directly into nearby streams or rivers and people use this water from the same source for domestic activities and also to wash slaughtered meat (Adeyemo, 2002; Akinro et al., 2009; Bello and Oyedemi, 2009). Often, contaminated water is used for crop irrigation and as drinking water for cattle and other habitants which indirectly causes pollution of the soil and jeopardizes human and

allow the construction of large lagoons (Johns, 1995). The lagoon processes have currently been improved in terms of reducing odour and offering potential of biogas utilisation. The concept of covering anaerobic lagoons has been developed. The covered anaerobic lagoons have been successfully applied to a range of industrial and abattoir wastewater demonstrating their cost effectiveness.

The most used form of anaerobic treatment process for domestic wastewater in Nigeria is the septic tank (Omenka, 2010). A septic tank is a self-contained, underground wastewater treatment system usually with two or more compartments. Septic refers to the anaerobic condition which develops in the tank. The effluent produced from a house consisting usually of blackwater (toilet waste) flows directly through the sewer pipe into the septic tank usually made of concrete or fibreglass. The septic tank is for pre-treatment and treats the wastewater by holding it in the tank with a retention time long enough for solids and liquids to separate. A septic tank removes many of the settleable solids, oils, greases, and floating debris in the raw wastewater. The removal efficiency of a septic tank that treats black water was studied in Bayelsa State of Nigeria and the result showed 54% BOD, 57% COD and 40% SS removal (Burubai et al., 2007).

There have been many reports of incidences of system failure and poor performances associated with septic tanks and associated soil water infiltration systems (Carrol et al., 2006). The poor performances of these systems are related with designs and site conditions not being properly investigated before the systems are sited (Dawes and Goonetilleke, 2003). In most cities in Nigeria, septic tanks are connected to soil water infiltration system for individual buildings including abattoirs. The infiltration system is mainly a pit with the sides used as infiltration surface. These pits are called soakaway pits and are connected directly to the septic tanks. Most of them are designed without following standards resulting to overflows or leaks causing a visible damage to the environment such as fishes in nearby streams (Burubai et al., 2007). This can also result to invisible groundwater pollution. Invisible groundwater pollution is actually a more serious problem since it will affect water supply and public health for decades (Sangodoyin and Agbawhe, 1992).

Thus, a process of identifying the appropriate treatment options for treating the effluents is of a high priority, since most abattoirs without treatment facilities are expected to continue discharging their sewage into the nearby rivers and agricultural drains. According to Omenka (2010), there are several technologies that can be used in conjunction with septic tanks; these technologies will help to effectively remove many contaminants before being discharged to the groundwater. Such systems include the intermittent sand filter, the soil water infiltration surface (bed, trenches, and mound) and constructed wetlands. The processes that take place in the intermittent filters include filtration or straining of suspended solids, sedimentation, biological process such as BOD removal and nitrification. Chemical adsorption of phosphorus can occur based on the media used such as activated carbon. An improvement to the intermitted sand filter is the multi-media anaerobic filtration tank which can perform treatment processes just as the intermittent sand filter and may assist in the production of methane for energy.

The objective of this paper is to investigate the potentiality of combining a septic and multi-media anaerobic filtration tanks to provide an efficient and economical treatment of abattoir waste.

2. Materials and Methods

Experimental Site

The investigation was conducted in Akure the capital city of Ondo–State. It is located in South Western Nigeria. The state has eighteen (18) local government areas and a land area of 13,595 km^2. Ondo State lies between longitudes 7^0 15'0"N and 5^{0}11'42 E of the Greenwich meridian. This means that the state lies entirely in the tropics. The temperature averages around 35^{0}C during the irrigation period.

Seven abattoirs within Akure were identified out of which four were selected for investigation of the physicochemical and microbiological properties of the effluent. For discussion, the abattoirs are identified as ARA located at Araromi, OBA located at Obanla, TOP located at Oluwatuyi and IYA located at FUTA junction (Table 1). The selected abattoirs were categorized under grade E abattoir with less than 10 slaughter units according to CISR technical guide K86 of Institute for Water Research. The method of killing cattle in these abattoirs is the traditional method of slaughtering at the slaughter slab after inspection by the health officers. Deep wells are the source of water supply for these abattoirs. Carcasses are cut up and sold to prospective buyers in the abutting meat shops. Waste generated in the abattoir include: bones, blood and dung. Dung is piled up and waste water containing blood and dung are discharged into a nearby stream without treatment. This results into pollution of surface and underground water especially of the abattoir and residents in the abattoir vicinity. Bones and hooves collected in the abattoir are burnt at the abattoir site causing smoke and air pollution. One major concern is that the abattoirs are surrounded with residential developments and office complexes. Other relevant information gathered from the investigation is summarized in Table 2.

Table 1: List of abattoirs and their location

Serial no	Name of Abattoir	Location	Ownership	Code
1	Araromi Abattoir	Araromi,	Public	ARA
2	Obanla Abattoir	Obanla	Public	OBA
3	Toplad Abattoir	Olukayode Street	Private	TOP
4	Iya ibeji Abattoir	FUTA junction	Private	IYA

Table 2: Some features of abattoirs under investigation

Features	Abattoir code			
	ARA	OBA	TOP	IYA
Years of operation	25 years	15years	5 years	3 years
cattle slaughter per day	20	10	5	2
Source of water	Chlorinated water Well water	Well water	Well water	Well water
Distance of abattoir to neighbouring streams	500 m	10 m	15 m	None

Distance between abattoir and nearest residential area	50 m	30 m	60 m	30 m
Nuisance posed by the waste	Flies, odour, Mosquitoes	Flies, odour,	Flies, odour , Mosquitoes	Flies, odour, Mosquitoes
Method of waste treatment	None	None	Screening	None
Point of discharge of effluent	Streams	Streams	Streams	Bush
Slaughter infrastructure	Concrete slab	Concrete slab	Concrete slab	Concrete slab
Use of receiving streams	Domestic, washing and irrigation			
Surface area the abattoir	12,000 m^2	8,500 m^2	400 m^2	300 m^2

Sampling method

Samples of abattoir wastewater were retrieved by grab sampling from the discharge pipe leading to the storage pond/septic tank of all the four abattoirs. Liquid samples were collected in a 1-liter bottle in triplicates for every sampling time and dates and stored at 4 °C between July and December 2005. Samples were collected every hour between 9.00a.m and 3.00 p.m. to make eighteen samples at the end of each day of sampling. The quality of wastewater sample varied with sampling time related to process occurring in the facility and the average of each parameter is determine for the day. The preserved sample were analysed in each case using Standard Methods recommended by American Public Health Association (APHA, 2005). The physical parameters analysed were pH, electrical conductivity, salinity, turbidity, TDS and TSS using colorimetric method. The chemical analyses performed were Dissolved Oxygen (DO), soluble COD (SCOD) after filtration on 0.45µm membrane filter, total COD (TCOD), oil and grease, nitrate- nitrogen, TKN and total phosphorus using colorimetric method. The HACH spectrophotometer DR2400 was used to read the concentrations. Temperature was measured with mercury thermometer immediately after sample collection.

Table 2 presents the composition of the raw wastewater prior to treatment except for the screening or settling of the coarse solids. It also shows that the strength of raw wastewater varies among abattoir depending on the size and type of ownership of each abattoir. Result of the analysis shows that OBA abattoir has the highest concentration of the physicochemical properties. It also shows that the Total COD, suspended solid (SS), total nitrogen (TKN), and total phosphorus (p) concentration of the raw wastewater collected at the four abattoirs are 2 to 9 times higher than a strong domestic wastewater which has a total COD of 1000mg/L, a SS content of 350mg/L, and TKN and P concentration of 85 and 5mg/L, respectively (Metcalf and Eddy, 2003). The abattoir wastewater generation was examined and information was collected on plant capacity, waste disposal, and water usage. To estimate the wastewater volume, the surveys were done to measure the quantity of blood lost per head killed in case of cattle, goat, and sheep. The bleeding time was about 7 minutes. For cattle, the average blood loss per head killed is 8 litters and 12 litres of paunch per head, and 20 litres and 6 litres in case of goat and sheep. Assuming 100% of water consumed by the abattoir becomes wastewater, the annual wastewater was estimated. Table 3 presents the quantity of wastewater produced. The total of wastewater per year was calculated considering wastewater from cattle, sheep and goat plus the annual water consumption. The means of data obtained from counts and physicochemical analysis were compared using one-way analysis of variance (ANOVA) in SPSS package. The coefficient of correlation between some physicochemical parameters was calculated by Pearson correlation test. Statistical significance was set at $p < 0.05$.

Table 3: Analysis of raw wastewater from four abattoirs prior to any treatment

Parameters	ARA(mg/l)	TOP(mg/l)	OBA(mg/l)	IYA(mg/l)
COD total	4976	2333	9665	3589
COD soluble	2817	778	4551	2605
Total solids	3862	2747	6037	2727
Volatile solids	3153	1204	4745	1966
Suspended solids	1348	877	2397	736
Volatile suspended solids	1192	594	2182	576
Total kjeldahl nitrogen	372	90	629	271
Ammonia	99	19	185	154
Protein	272	71	444	117
Total phosphorous	0	28	61	0
PH	7.2	6.5	6.8	6.7

3. Design and Operation of the Treatment Unit

Design consideration

In waste treatment technology, the goal of a designer is to promote the simplest treatment scheme available that will meet the requirements of the permit while providing maximum ease of operation. Cost comparisons and long term operability are also very important. In designing this unit, the objective was to design a low cost, simple, efficient and easy-to-operate treatment technology whereby using the existing facilities in the abattoirs. The construction material for the treatment unit was expected to be sourced locally and generally available. This technology was expected to follow the treatment train as highlighted in the literature review. Of most importance was the consideration of a treatment process that goes beyond the level of conventional treatment processes of the removal of COD and suspended solid to removal of significant amounts of nitrogen, phosphorus, heavy metals, biodegradable organics and also odour and colour. A combination of a wedge-wire screen, a two compartment septic tank and a filtration tank using activated carbon was proposed. A Typical treatment plant flowchart incorporating all these processes is illustrated in Figure 1.

Figure 1: The flowchart for treatment plant

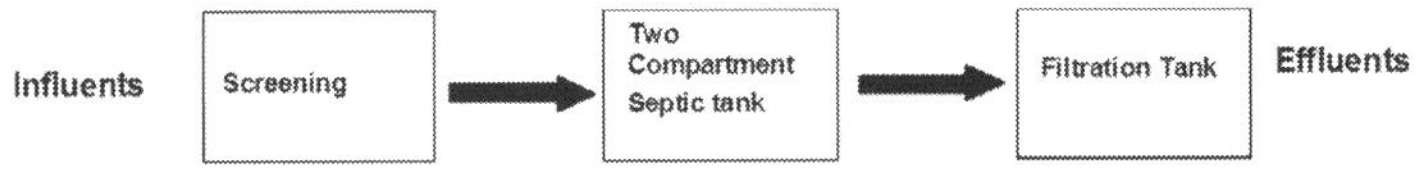

Looking at the flowchart (see Figure 1), preliminary treatment was provided by screening. The screening was expected to remove gross pollutants from the effluent streams so as to protect the downstream equipments from damage or overloading. Obanla abattoir was selected for trial because of the cost of production of replicate of treatment plant. It was also considered as the most suitable for the experiment due its highest concentration of the raw wastewater composition. In Obanla abattoir, a septic tank already existed but it was later modified into a two compartment septic tank, which acts as the primary/

secondary treatment using anaerobic process of biological treatment. The first compartment provided sedimentation, sludge digestion and sludge storage. The second compartment provided additional sedimentation and sludge- storage capacity and thus served to protect against the discharge of sludge and other materials that might escape through the first chamber (Metcalf and Eddy 2003). The factors that were considered before the design of the treatment plants are; 1) the area of the wire mesh and the hole diameter; 2) Grade and requirements of abattoir under consideration; 3) Volume of the sewerage water; 4) Loading condition ; 5)Capacity of Septic tank; 6) Location of the septic tank; 7) Inlet, outlet and inter-compartment arrangements; 8) Volume of the filter medium and 9) Depth, diameter and uniformity coefficient of media.

Septic Tank Design

Since all the abattoirs in Akure were categorized under grade E abattoir with less than 10 slaughter units according to CISR technical guide K86 of Institute for Water research. It was stipulated that abattoirs would require a water supply of at least 900 litres per slaughter unit and it is expected that the volume of effluent is an approximate of 80-85% of water required. A two compartments septic tank is expected to have a minimum capacity of 130% of total daily sewage flow for first compartment and at least 20% of total daily sewage flow for second compartment. Following the calculations, a 9000liters capacity tank was designed to cater for a Grade E abattoir which has between 1–8 slaughter units (Figure 4). Polyvinyl chloride (PVC) pipe tube and hose (internal diameter=1m) were used for influent and effluents distribution. A retention value was installed at the influents entrance to prevent sludge from flowing out during maintenance operation. After treatment, the effluent collected from the second compartment of the septic tank is later pumped to the anaerobic filtration tank. The design calculation is as follow:

(i) *Volume of the sewerage water*

For a grade E Abattoir with a maximum of 8 slaughtering unit =

8 X 900

= 7200 litres

Considering 80% of water as effluents =

7200 * 0.80

= 5760 litres

(ii) Capacity of septic tank

Considering 130% of the sewerage water for first compartment =

5760* 130%

= 7450 litres.

For 20% of sewerage for 2 compartment =

5760* 20%

= 1152

Therefore total capacity of Tank =

7450 + 1152

8602 litres ~ 9000 litres.

The Anaerobic filter design

The anaerobic filters (AF) as earlier discussed act as an attached growth or fixed film reactor. It is a column filled with various types of media. Such media are sand, coarse gravel, pea gravel and activated carbon. The treatment process was done by passing the liquid through sand /carbon arrayed as a porous media in columns or beds. Removal by filtration includes two steps: particle transport and attachment. Once attachment has occurred, a biofilm developed on the sand grains of a sand bed may metabolize organic contaminants, resulting in permanent removal. The transport mechanisms include interception, sedimentation, and diffusion. As wastewater passes through an intermittent sand filter, several mechanisms act to filter out and chemically change both suspended solids and dissolved materials found in the wastewater. Two filtering actions are involved: 1) the physical removal of suspended matter by straining, adsorption and sedimentation on the downstream side of the sand grain and 2) the biochemical removal of colloidal and dissolved organic substances which are transformed into stable materials (Metcalf and Eddy, 2003; US EPA, 2002). Apart from the physical separation of suspended solids and additional reduction of COD, the activated carbon media in the filter was to further remove the odour and colour of the wastewater. A schematic diagram of the anaerobic filter is shown in Figure 5.

A transparent plastic container was initially constructed as prototypes to test run the experiment prior to the design of the filter unit (Figure 2b). The filters was first filled with 5 cm layer of pea gravel to ensure proper drainage which is followed by 40 cm layer of fine sand layer which was overlaid with 20 cm of activated carbon and 20cm of coarse sand . The filter was lastly sealed with a 20mm layer of pea gravel on the surface. The sand was washed before use to remove clay and other mineral contaminants from the sand particles.The pea gravel has an effective diameter range of 3.80mm and uniformity coefficient of 1.68, while course sand has an effective diameter range of 1.35 and uniformity coefficient of 1.68 and the fine sand with effective diameter range of 0.93mm and uniformity coefficient of 1.50 while activated charcoal has an effective diameter of 0.52mm and uniformity coefficient of 1.80 (Figure 2a and 2b). The filtrates were collected at the basement of the filtration tank for further test after 2 or 3 days.

Design Considerations

Design parameters that were considered are:

1. Grain size and uniformity: The effectiveness of the granular material as filter media is related to the size, uniformity, and composition of the grains. The size of the granular media correlates with the surface area available to support the microorganisms that treat the wastewater (US EPA, 2002).

2. Depth of a filter: For design parameters of intermittent sand filter, criteria generally recommend a depth of 60 to 90 cm (24 to 36 inches) (US EPA, 2002).

3. Multi layered structure: Literature shows that multiple layer sand filters had better BOD_5 and COD removal than single lay-

er sand filters. A three-layer sand filter had the highest COD removal capacity due to longer filter runs. The coarser top layer of sand filter was used as pre-treatment of wastewater with high concentration of active biomass and sufficient O_2 supply (Liu et al, 1999), protecting the finer lower layers from clogging at higher loading rates (Venhuizen, 1996).

4. Hydraulic loading rate: Since bacteria removal is most effective through the upper part of filter, faster flow caused by larger dosing volume may result in lower removal. Larger doses lead to less time available for diffusion of bacteria into the less mobile fraction of pore water resulting in less effective adsorption processes in the top area of the sand filter. If the daily dosing rate needs to be increased, an increased frequency of doses would be preferred rather than increasing the dose size (Stevik et al., 1999).

5. Distribution methods:Equal distribution of the wastewater over the whole filter surface has benefit with respect to water as well as air transport (Schudel and Boller, 1990). Localized overloading caused by poor distribution of wastewater over the filters may result in intermittent or continuous saturated flow and probable poor purification performance (Converse et al., 1974).

Figure 2a and 2b show the picture and schematic design of the bench-scale multi-media filter respectively

Figure 2a **Figure 2b**

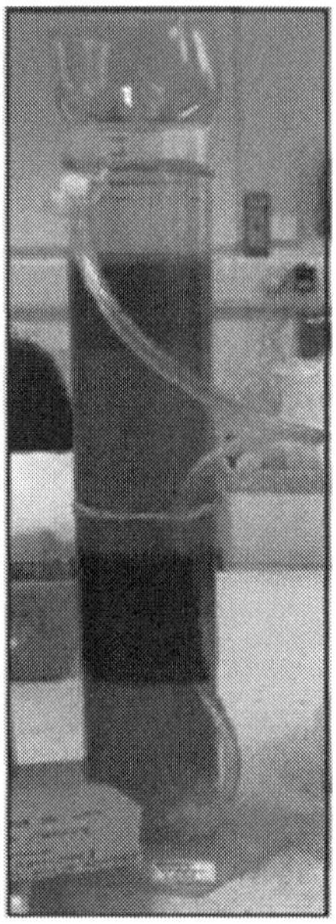

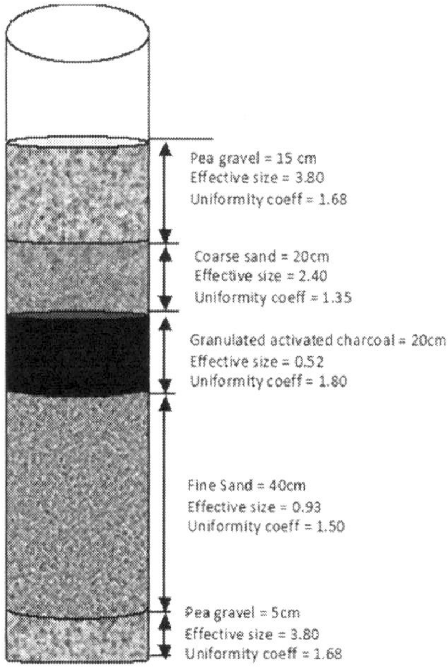

The design calculation is as follows:

(i) Volume of filter medium

The volume required for the mediums are as calculated below:

Assuming the Area of the filter unit is to be $0.25m^2$ (Figure 3), the volume of 20cm of pea gravel medium is calculated as

$0.25m^2 \times 0.2m = 0.05m^3$

$0.05 \times 1000 = 50$ litres.

The total volume considering 20cm layer of pea gravel , activated carbon and course gravel will be 150 litres and in addition to 40cm layer of fine sand. Therefore the total volume is

$50+50+50+100 = 250$ litres.

Given that filter capacity is 250 litres = length x breath x depth.

Depth = $0.25m^3/0.25m^2$

Depth = 1m

(ii) Calculating the storage depth

Assuming filtrate volume of ≥200 litres

Therefore volume =

1 x b x d

200 litres = 0.5 x 0.5 x d

Therefore

$0.2m^3$ = 0.25 x d

d = 0.2/0.25

Depth = 0.8m

Figure 3: Area of the tank

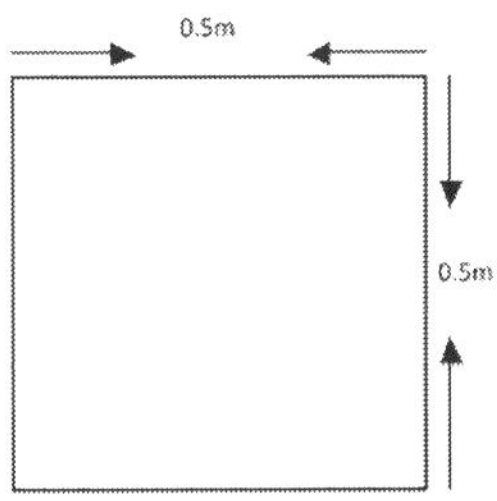

Height of filtrations tank = filter depth + storage depth =

1 + 0.8= 1.8m.

(iii) The Strainer's outlet

Length of strainer plate= 0.5m

Breath of strainer plate= 0.5m

Diameter of strainer hole= 0.002m

Inter hole spacing= 0.010m

Intra hole spacing= 0.010m

Surface area of strainer plate =

0.5 x 0.5 = $0.25m^2$

No. of holes to be drilled across the length of strainer will be inter hole spacing + hole diameter

= 0.010 + 0.002

= 0.012m

Therefore No of holes = length / (spacing + hole diameter)

= 0.5 / 0.012

= 42 holes

Since the strainer plate is square and the inter row and intra row spacing are the same, the number of holes across the length is the same across the breath which is 42 holes.

Total number of straining holes

= 42 x 42

= 1746 holes

Area of holes = $(d^2 / 4)$ x 1746 holes

= x 0.00022 x 1746 / 4 Inter row spacing 0.010m

= 0.0055m2

If the surface area is $0.25m^2$ and the area of holes is $0.0055m^2$, and the

Area of holes is $0.0055m^2$, therefore

Area of space left = 0.25 - 0.0055

= $0.2445m^2$

= $0.24m^2$

(iv) Design of spray shower

The spray shower that loads the water into the filtrations tank has a diameter of 0.08m and a set diameter of 0.001m. Since it has to spray the water evenly across the surface areas, it had to be raised to a height taking into consideration the angle at which the shower sprays downwards.

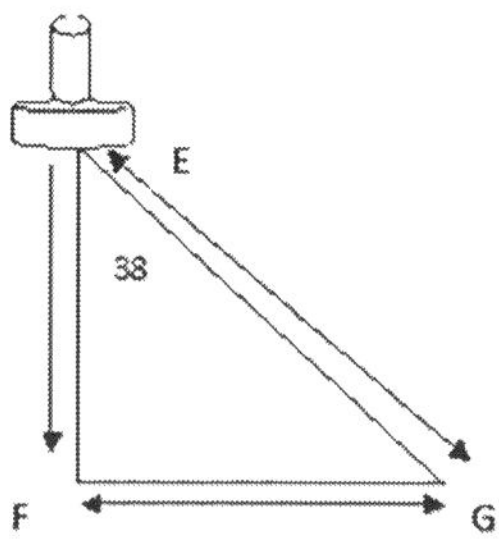

Ab = 0.5

Ad = 0.5

From Pythagoras theorem

Ac = $(ad^2 + dc2)$ ½

Ac = 0.707

The angle at which the shower sprays downwards was gotten to be 38^0

Figure is half of ac = 0.3535

From trigonometry

Tan 38^0 = fg / ef

Where ef is the height of the spray shower from the center of the filtrations tank surface.

$Ef = fg / Tan\ 38^0$

$Ef = 0.3535 / 0.7812$

$Ef = 0.45m$

The height of the shower from the filtrations tank surface will be 0.45m. Since the height is 0.45m from the surface, the rod holding the shower that is inclined at 38⁰ will have a length of:

$Eg = (ef^2 + fg^2)1/2$

$Eg = (0.45^2 + 0.3535^2)\ ½$

$Eg = 0.57m$

An additional allowance for proper setting was added to the rod to give 0.60m four of such rods where used to hold the shower and four hollow pipes of internal diameter 8mm and external diameter 10mm were also used to hold the shower stand to the tank internally at the top. To hold the strainer plate inside the tank, an angle iron of 0.02m by 0.02m with a thickness of 0.004m was used inside the filtration tank.

Figure 4 and Figure 5 show schematic diagrams of a 9000 litres two-compartment septic tank and anaerobic filtration tank respectively.

Figure 4: Schematic diagram of a 9000 litres two-compartment septic tank

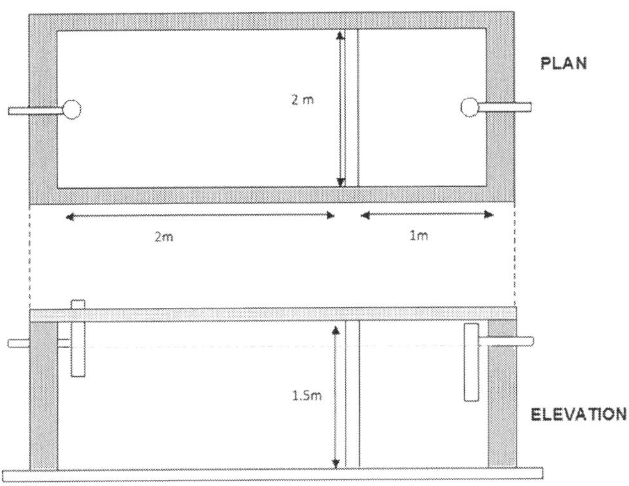

Figure 5: Schematic diagram of anaerobic filtration tank

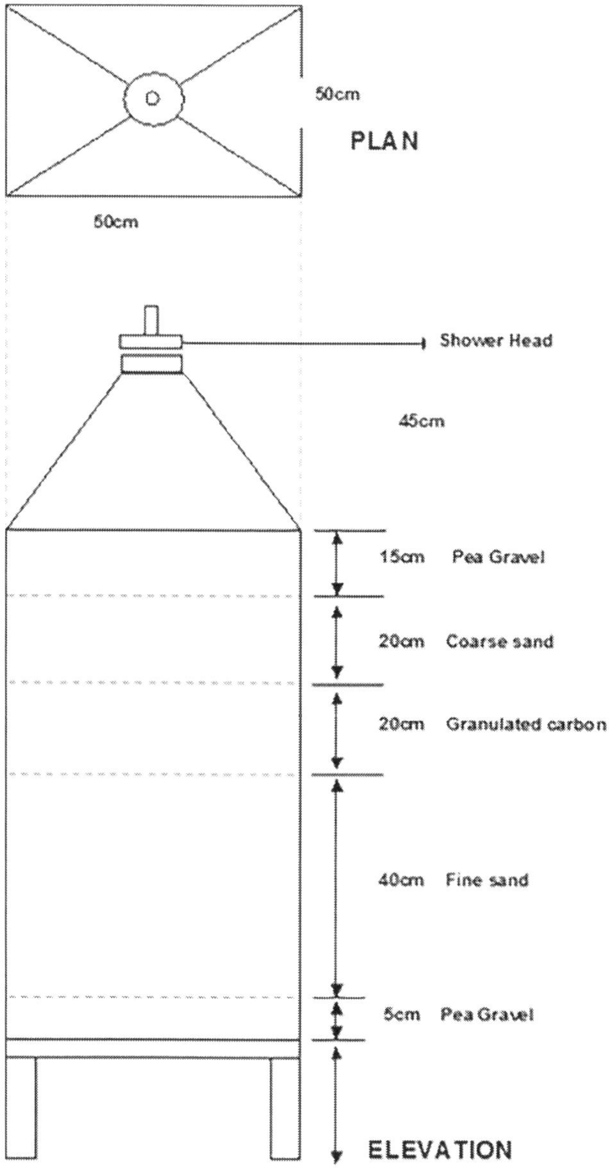

4. Results and Discussion

The startup period was monitored and the effluents were allowed to have a dentition period of 40 days in the septic tank before it was later pumped to the filtration tank. Table 4 gives the average concentrations of total and soluble COD, solids and nutrients of influents fed to the treatment plants before and after treatment.

Table 4: Quality of wastewater from OBA abattoir before and after treatments

Parameters	Influents (mg/l)	Effluent after leaving the septic tank	Removal (%)	Final Effluents (mg/l)	Removal (%)
COD total	9665	4217	56	2108	78
COD soluble	4551	2146	53	1120	75
Total solids	6037	2765	54	3381	44
Volatile solids	4745	3134	33	1406	70
Suspended solids	2397	1570	35	460	81
Volatile suspended solids	2182	2183	0	810	63
Total kjeldahl nitrogen	629	596	5	552	12
Ammonia	185	**	**	512	-177
Protein	444	120	73	33	93
Total phosphorous	61	61	0	59	2
PH	6.8	7.0	0	7.2	0
Methane(m^3/kg of VS fed)	0	0.54-0.61			

From the investigations, the result obtained as shown in Table 4 compared to Table 3 highlights the level of removal of these compounds most especially the reduction in COD. A high COD removal was achieved in the total and soluble COD, which reduces from 9665mg/l and 4551mg/l to 2108mg/l and 1120mg/l respectively. The percentage reduction of 78% and 75% shows that the removal efficiency of the treatment plant is very high, indicating that the technology is very stable and efficient. The reduction was due to microbial activities in the septic tank. The results also show that both the Septic and Filtration Tanks had excellent settling characteristics even though the quiescent conditions were sometimes disturbed by biogas production. The removal of the COD total, COD soluble and suspended solids by 56%, 53% and 35% respectively by the septic tank is in agreement with the report from Bayesa, Nigeria (Burubai et al, 2007). The septic tank also has a maximum removal of protein of 444mg/l to 120mg/l resulting to 73% reduction in protein. This is as result of bio-dragration of protein into energy under the anaerobic condition. This can be correlated with the high production of 0.54-0.6 m^3/kg of VS fed for Methane. The methane production is high compared to 0.52 - 0.55m^3/kg of VS and 0.22 m3/kg of VS as reported by Salminen et al., (2000) and Safley et al. (1987). This can be attributed to the climatic condition in Akure and due to minimum pre-treatment of the waste before getting into the septic tank. When observing the removal rate of the final effluent after further treatment with the multi-media anaerobic filtration tanks, the TS, VS, SS and VSS concentration in the effluents with initial concentration of 6037, 4745mg/l 2397mg/l and 2182mg/l were reduced to 3381mg/l, 1406mg/l, 460mg/l and 810mg/l having a percentage removal of 44% for TS, 70% for VS, 85% for SS and 63% for VSS respectively. The final reduction is as a result of the technology involved in the treatments of the wastewater which include various numbers of filter media and the inclusion of activated carbon for the adsorption process. The filtrate showed a significant reduction in the odour and colour compared to raw slaughter house wastewater. Also, the dark colouration of raw effluents had completely disappeared and the treated wastewater has turned to a pale yellowish colour. The changes in the odour and the colour were as a result of the adsorption capacity of the activated carbon. This can be characterized by the adsorption that occurs when components of a liquid (the poison) attaches to a solid (activated carbon). This can be either physical or chemical in nature, and can frequently involve both.

The removal of Total kjeldahl nitrogen is by 15% and this is in agreement with Metcalf and Eddy 2003. Since nitrogen is an essential building block in the production of protein, the predominance of nitrogen is an indication that the wastewater has been stabilised with respect to oxygen demand. The nitrate is being used by algae and other aquatic plants to form plant protein. The removal of the nitrogen will reduce the biological process of waste treatment. Also, phosphorus is also essential to growth of algae and other biological organisms that aid in the treatment in the septic tank (biological processes). Therefore the removal of nitrogen to this extent using a biological process in the secondary treatment shows that the treatment processes are still very efficient.

The effluents had an average value of PH 7.2, which is slightly higher than the influent; this is as a result of the reaction in the treatment plant. This will increase the buffering capacity of the wastewater, thus beneficial. Lastly, the high degree of mechanization compared to high COD removed is an indication that the wastewater was effectively degraded.

5. Economic Analysis

The economic analysis of abattoir wastewater treatment plant was based on the costs and benefits of the treatment unit. The economic costs for the system was based on the capital cost (design, purchase and installation costs) and running costs (operation and maintenance). A summary of the capital and operating and maintenance (O&M) costs for the plant is shown in Table 5. In general, the cost of the filtration tank and the modification of the septic tank drove the capital costs of the project. The capital cost is about ₦175, 000 consisting of civil works on the septic tank and cost of equipment and installations of the filtration tank. This budget was based on the assumption that the septic tank was newly constructed even though an existing septic tank was modified. The annual running cost of operating the plant was estimated to be ₦140, 600 as shown in Table 5. This includes cost items such as manpower and electricity. The electricity consumption was calculated based on continuous 24-hr operation and a power cost of 5₦/Kw-h. The total annual power cost of the plant was calculated at about ₦57600 per year. The manpower item was calculated for one technician (at ₦2000 per month). It is clear from design that the power usage in the plant is only consumed in the feed pump attached to the filtration tank. There were no chemicals used in the treatment therefore it was no estimated but the water quality analysis was estimated to be ₦59, 000. Some of the economic benefits considered as a result of the treatment unit is the sale of cow dung after screening. The cow dung is mostly sold to the public or the state waste management authority for the production of organic fertilizer and it was estimated to be about ₦10 per kg (Ipinmoroti et al 2009) and considering an average of 10 cows slaughtered per day. On average, a full-grown cow produces approximately 150 Lbs or 68Kg of manure per day; therefore, the cost of cow dung is estimated to be ₦6, 800 per day and about ₦1.77million per year excluding weekends. Assuming half of cow dung is sold daily, the total benefit from cow dung per year is estimated to be ₦885,000. The biogas production was also roughly estimated based on the land covered by the septic tank and it was estimated to be ₦165, 000 per year. The environmental benefit was not expressed in monetary terms in the report but can be considered for future work. Also, the land used for the unit was not put in consideration because a septic tank already existed before the research was conducted and the total area covered by the filtration tank is negligible. The cost benefit ratio was calculated as 3.33, which indicates a profitability of the system. In general, the purpose of these economic considerations is to demonstrate that the process is potentially, economically competitive with existing technologies and to illustrate which factors drive cost.

Table 5: Economic analysis of the treatment unit at OBA abattoir

Item		Cost(N)	Cost ($)
Capital Cost	Civil work (Construction of Septic tank)	55,000.00	366.67
	Equipment Cost	50,000.00	333.33
	Equipment Installation	70,000.00	466.67
	Total Capital Cost	**175,000.00**	**1,166.67**
Operation and maintenance (O&M) Cost	Manpower	24,000.00	160.00
	Water Quality test	59,000.00	393.33
	Power cost	57,600.00	384.00
	Total annual running cost	**140,600.00**	**937.33**
	Total Economic Cost	**315,600.00**	**2,104.00**
Benefit	Biogas production	165,000.00	1,100.00
	Sale of Cow Dung	885,000.00	5,900.00
	Total benefit	**1,050,000.00**	**7,000.00**
	Benefit/Cost ratio	**3.33**	**3.33**

6. Conclusion

The preliminary data of the filtration tank samples show that the proposed technology has good potential to substantially reduce the pollution load of the slaughterhouse effluents. The filtrate shows significant reduction in odour and colour. The digested effluents were almost odourless when compared to the biomass. The septic tank also provided good solids-liquid separation. The proposed process has a good potential to provide the abattoir industry with a more environmentally sound wastewater management alternative. It will eliminate the need for expensive air flotation and sedimentation process currently used for treating abattoir wastewater. Finally, the above process can be used to recover a significant quantity of energy (methane) that could be used to heat or produce hot water at the abattoir plant.

References

Akinro, A. O., Ologunagba, I. B. and Olotu Y. (2009), 'Environmental implications of unhygienic operation of a city abattoir in Akure, Western Nigeria', in *Journal of Engineering and Applied Sciences,* 4(9): 1819-6608.

Adeyemo, O. K. (2002), 'Unhygienic operation of a city abattoir in south western Nigeria: environmental implication', in *AJEAM/RAGEE*, 491: 23-28.

APHA, (2005), 'Standard Methods for the Examination of Water and Wastewater', in*American Public Health Association /American Water Works Association/Water Environment Federation*, Washington D.C.

Batstone, D., Keller, J., Newell, B. and Newland, M. (1997), 'Model development and full scale validation for anaerobic treatment of protein and fat based wastewater', in *Water Science and Technology*, 36: 423–431.

Bello, Y. O. and Oyedemi, D.T.A. (2009), 'The Impact of abattoir activities and management in residential neighbourhoods: a case study of Ogbomoso', in *Nigeria Journal of Social Science*, 19(2): 121-127.

Burubai, W., Akor, A.J., Lilly, M.T., and Ayawari D.T. (2007), 'An evaluation of septic tank performance in Bayelsa State, Nigeria', in*Agricultural Engineering International: The CIGR Ejournal*, 19:1-9.

Carroll, S., Goonetilleke, A., and Thomas, E., (2006), 'Integrated risk framework for onsite wastewater treatment system' in*Environmental Management Journal*, 38(2): 286-303.

Converse, J. C., Anderson, J. L., Ziebell, W. A. and J. Bouma. (1974), 'Pressure distribution of improving Soil adsorption systems' in *Proceedings of National Symposium Home Sewage Disposal, ASAE*: 104-116.

Dawes, L. and Goonetilleke, A. (2003), 'An investigation into the role of site and soil characteristics in onsite sewage treatment', in *Journal of Environmental Geology*, 44(4): 467 -477.

Environmental Protection Agency, (EPA) (2002), 'Development document for the proposed effluent limitations guidelines and standards for the meat and poultry products industry point source category', *EPA-821-B-01-007*, Cincinnati, OH, Office of Water.

Ipinmoroti R.R., Iremiren, G. O., Olubamiwa, O., Fademi, A.O. and Aigbekaen, E.O. (2009), 'Effect of inorganic and organic based fertilizers on growth performance of tea and cost implication in Kusuku, Nigeria' in *Proceedings of 9th African Crop Science-Conference*, Cape Town, South Africa, 27th September – 2nd October, 2009.

Johns, M.R. (1995), 'Developments in wastewater treatment in the meat processing industry: a review', in *Bioresource Technology*, 54: 203–216.

Liu, Q., Mancl, K. M. and Tuovinen, O. H. (1999), 'Study of the use of fine media biofilm reactors to renovate high fat wastewater', in *Small Flows Journal*, 5(1): 4-11.

Marriott, N.G. (1999), '*Principles of food sanitation*,' Aspen, Gaithersburg, MD, USA, pp 364.

Massé, D.I. and Masse, L. (2000), 'Characterization of wastewater from hog slaughterhouses in Eastern Canada and evaluation of their in-plant wastewater treatment system', in *Canadian Agricultural Engineering Journal*, 42(3):139-146.

Mata-Alvarez, J. (2003), '*Biomethanization of organic fraction of municipal solidwastes*', *IWA* publishing. ISBN: 1 900222140

Metcalf, X. and Eddy, X. (2003), '*Wastewater engineering: treatment, disposal and reuse*', McGraw-Hill, New York, Fourth Edition, p. 1848.

Muhirwa, D, Nhapi, I. and Rulinda, J.B. (2006), 'Characterization of abattoir wastewater of Kigali', in *Proceedings of 3rd International Conference on Appropriate Technology*, Kigali, Rwanda,November 12 – 15.

Omenka E. (2010), 'Improvement of decentralized wastewater treatment in Asaba, Nigeria', MSc *Thesis, Lund University*, Sweden.

Safley Jr. L.M., Vetter, R.L., Smith, D. (1987), 'Operating a full-scale poultry manure anaerobic digester', in *Biological Wastes*, 19: 79–90.

Salminen, E., Rintala, J., Lokshina, L.Y., Vavilin, V.A. (2000), 'Anaerobic batch degradation of solid poultry slaughterhouse waste', in *Water Science and Technology*, 41(3): 33–41.

Sangodoyin, A.Y and Agbawhe, O.M. (1992), 'Environmental study on surface and ground water pollutants from abattoir effluents', in *Bioresource Technology*, 41(3): 193-200.

Schudel, A. and Boller M. (1990), 'Onsite wastewater treatment with intermittent buried filters', in *Water Science and Technology*, 22(3/4): 93-100.

Skjelhaugen O. J. and Donantoni, L. (1998), 'Combined aerobic and electrolytic treatment of cattle slurry', in *Journal of Agricultural Engineering Research*, 70: 209–219.

Stevik, T. K., Ausland, G., Jenssen, P. D. and Siegrist, R. (1999), 'Removal of *E.coli* during intermittent filtration of wastewater effluent as affected by dosing rate and media type', in *Water Science and Technology*, 33: 2088-2098.

US-EPA, (2002), 'Environmental assessment of proposed effluent limitations guidelines and standards for the meat and poultry products industry point source,' *EPA-821-B-01008*, Office of Water, US Environmental Protection Agency, Washington, D.C.

Venhuizen, D. (1996), 'Intermittent sand filters: new frontiers for an ancient art'. Available at: http://klingon.util.utexas.edu/VenhSandFilter/VenhSandFilter.html.

Chapter 4

Community View of Public Water Projects and the Challenges Posed to State Institutions in Nigeria

Emmanuel M. Akpabio

1. Introduction

The search for effective water management options in local communities generally overlooks beliefs systems, perception, environmental reality and attitudes. Yet these all play a part in sustainable water resources management most especially in the less developed Countries. For instance, how do tradition and religion affect peoples' notions of water? What determines rights of access to water as well as management practices in such context? These and related questions constitute the core of traditional ecological worldview of water resources management in Africa. Such worldviews depend on a number of factors including historical, geographical and cultural contexts. Linton (2010) observed that people inhabiting deserts have tended to form ideas (and metaphors) that differ markedly from those formed by people living in humid regions. The author went on to say that all ideas of water are hybrids in the sense that they are at once social and natural, internalizing the emergent-that is, historical and geographical-properties of H_20 along with historical and geographical circumstances of the thinker. Groenfeldt (1991), while looking at the various irrigation practices in Asia, came to the conclusion that the physical properties of water alone do not determine a homogenous social response. According to the author, the solutions to these universal problems are 'unique to each indigenous system, depending upon the particular social and cultural traditions, the particular physical setting, and the particular individuals concerned'. In another instance, Sokile and Van Koppen (2004) observed that in sub-Saharan Africa, water is the basis for life for agro-and for pastoral societies and its allocation mechanism is firmly tied to the deeper sociocultural and economic context that cannot be simply understood by mainstream economic, social, and legal principles. These imply that water is not only the natural stuff that one sees and uses but a social and cultural substance that forms the locus of interaction between humans and the non-human worlds. John Donahue and Barbara Rose Johnston (cited in Linton 2010: 58) highlighted the need to investigate the links between how water gets defined, how it gets managed, and for whose benefit: 'what different cultural meanings does water have for the contending parties, and how do these meanings complicate mediation among the various interests? How are some social actors able to impose their definition of water on other social actors with different but equally legitimate definitions? In other words, how is power used in the service of one or another of the cultural definitions of water?'

The way people perceive water shapes their attitudes to management. Based on this context, how do conventional water management paradigms fit into local perceptions and practices? What are the roles and challenges of state institutions in guaranteeing efficient, accountable and equitable management of water resources? These and related questions will be answered by looking at how modern water management principles such as water rights, cost recovery and sustainability principles of the state compares favorably with local practices within the Cross River Basin (CRB), Nigeria. The study pays particular emphasis on areas of commonalities and differences as well as exploring how areas of differences could be resolved. Project units of the Cross River Basin Development Authority (CRBDA) in Akwa Ibom state are used for analysis.

2. Brief Insight into the study area

The study was conducted in Akwa Ibom state, south-south Nigeria (between latitudes 4° 30′ N and 5° 30′ N and longitudes 7° 30′ E and 8° 15′ E) (Figure 1).

Figure 1: Akwa Ibom State with Approximate Water Levels

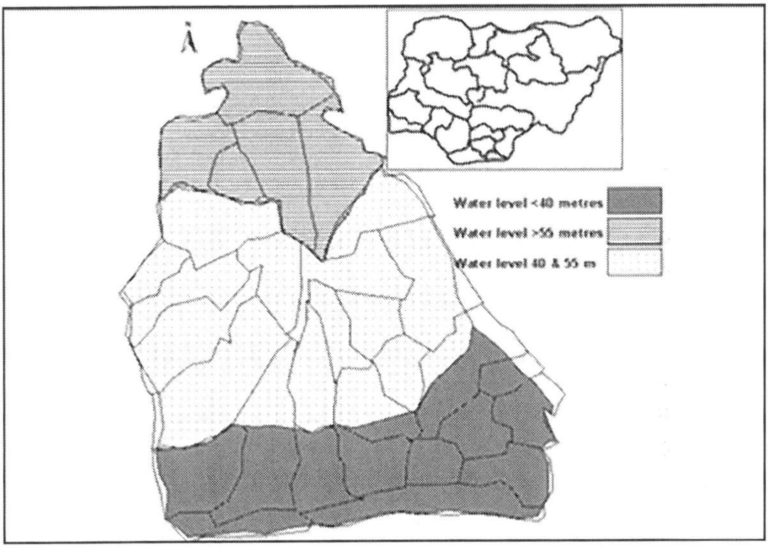

Based on soils and land use surveys (AKS, 1989), Akwa Ibom State is divided into 3 hydro geological areas based on the regional water table. They include: 1) South (Ikot Abasi, Eket and Oron Local government areas with water level accessible at less than 40 metres). The south happens to be an area dominated by onshore/offshore petroleum oil exploration with such major oil multinationals as Shell, Exon Mobil, Agip, Elf and Total oil, whose activities pose pollution problems to available sources of drinking water. It is also constantly washed by the southern Atlantic Ocean; 2) the middle (Uyo, Etinan, Abak, Essien Udim, Oruk Anam, among others) with a water level values ranging between 40 and 55 metres. As coastal plain sand, the lithology of the area is very favorable for the storage and extraction of groundwater. Consequently, private and commercial borehole engagement are very common in this region, especially taking advantage of high urban and consequent demographic growth; 3) and the North (Itu, Ini, Ikono, northern part of Ikot Ekpene Local Government Areas with the water level values greater than 55 meters). The northern boundary of the aquifer is formed by the impervious clays and shale of the Ameke and Imo shale formations (AKS, 1989). This geological condition makes it difficult for ground water extraction, and where such extraction is possible, there is the other problem of mineral-based water pollution. From these classifications, it is seen that water resources availability is highly variable across spatial areas. In general, the State is well endowed with vast resources of both surface and groundwater as annual rainfall ranges between 2000 mm and 3000mm, which occurs mainly between March and October of every year (AKS, 1989).

Akwa Ibom State has three major ethnic groups (namely, Ibibio, Annang and Oron) with a total population of 3,920,208 spread across a landmass of 8,412km^2 (NPC, 2007). Agriculture and related works are the main sources of livelihood and income activities for the rural populace while the rest of the economically employed population are mostly found in the urban areas (Ekong, 2003). Over ninety percent of Akwa Ibom indigenes are Christians, with a significant number subscribing to the new Pentecostal movement. The growing tendency towards the new Pentecostal movement reflect the faith and belief of the people in the spiritual solution to existential and livelihood problems. Traditional rulers, by the oath of their office, maintain traditional (pagan) form of worship, through libation and regular communication with ancestors. In general, there is a blending of some basic elements of the traditional and Christian beliefs, and the Christians most often respect and are subject to the traditional institutions of governance especially in the rural areas.

There are two sources of water supply in the state: the natural sources and the modern supply sources. The natural sources are still useful to a vast majority of the people especially in the rural areas. Availability is a matter of direct collection of rainwater in containers and extraction from streams, ponds and hand-dug wells. Although generally viewed as primitive, this system has its good points, especially the multi-source and self-reliant aspects. All the available local sources are used, depending on the people's perception of quality, seasonal availability and technological know-how (Faniran, 1981). Natural sources serve about 80%-90% of the state's population, which is predominantly rural. In most cases, the natural source of water is community based and community-driven. The modern supply sources started with the British during the colonial period. At best, the modern supply scheme is a public-sector affair, undertaken and maintained by government at public expense e.g., the water supply undertaken by the Akwa Ibom state water boards. Such schemes could be found in taps at public and private places. At worst, modern supply source is individually owned e.g. a private or commercial borehole. Customary water rights in the rural areas are mostly embedded in the land tenure system. Although, the system of land ownership also influences water rights, Akpabio (2005) however noted that in most communities there is a clear difference between land and water rights. This means one can have exclusive land rights but water bodies belong to the community, where everybody has the right of access. This practice is reinforced by traditional recognition of water bodies as God given (*Mmọ edi ake Abasi*), which implies that no single individual has exclusive right over water bodies - the context and basis for a collective management and control of available water resources.

The result of the study is based on the CRBDA projects, namely, Abak irrigation, Itu drainage and irrigation projects, Nkari earth dam as well as numerous community drinking water schemes set up by the basin authority. These projects were used since they form the intersection points between the CRBDA (as a state agent) and local communities. Village meetings, focus groups, interviews and researcher's past personal village experiences were important sources of field data. Issues that were given much attention during data collection include rights and access issues, cost recovery, equity and environmental sustainability, among others.

3. Current state water management instruments

The basis for Akwa Ibom State involvement in water resources management come from various sources such as legal, legislative and administrative at national, state and local levels. Constitutionally, water resource is placed in the concurrent list of the 1999 constitution, involving all tiers of government and private sector. Consequently, statutory rights to water resources are embedded in the Land Use Act of 1978 and Water resources decree of 1993. Other key regulatory and legal instruments with direct or indirect impact on water resources management are scattered in various other documents as listed in Table 1.

The provisions in the land Use Acts give individuals absolute rights to ground water resources through land rights while the water resources decree 101 of 1993 vests all matters of water rights in the federal government of Nigeria. The broad regulatory power of the government in connection with land and groundwater use may adversely affect customary rights. The Water Resources decree enables the government to define the times and manner at which water may be taken, prohibit the taking of water for health reasons or even revoke customary rights in the public interest. Similarly, under section 28 of the Land Use Act, any right of occupancy, including customary rights of occupancy, is subject to revocation for overriding public interest which is defined to include "the requirement of land for mining purposes or oil pipelines" or the requirement of land for public purposes by the Federal, state or local governments. However, it would be a mistake to assume in all cases that customary rights would always be subordinate to statutory rights. Significantly, under section 2 of the Water Resources decree, "any person may (i) take water without charge for his domestic purpose or for watering his livestock from any water course to which the public has free access; or (ii) may use water for the purpose of fishing or for navigation to the extent that such use is not inconsistent with any other law for the time being in force..." Because the term free access has not been defined, it is an open question whether the issue of access to water for domestic purposes should also be determined by taking into account customary law rights Kuruk, undated). To the extent customary law rules are relevant, potentially there could be a conflict between a user who claims a right to use water for domestic purposes under the Water Resources decree but which is resisted by a community group that claims to restrict access under their customary rules (mostly linked to cultural factors). It is unclear in this case how the issue will ultimately be resolved. These factors were observed to play out in the implementation of water resources programs and projects in Akwa Ibom state and they form the nucleus of discussions in this paper. My discussions on these factors will draw on the concept of 'common resources' and attempt to link it with indigenous notions of water resources. The goal will be to see how such notions have enhanced or undermined the workings of relevant state institutions in the implementation of water resources programs in Akwa Ibom state.

Table 1: Water Resources Related Management Instruments in Nigeria

S/N	Name of Statutes	Key provisions
1	The Waterworks Act of 1915	Colonial Nigeria (shortly after Amalgamation in 1914) passed the law specifically to keep water from being polluted. It prohibits the pollution of water in Nigeria by obnoxious or harmful matters.
2	Nigerian Minerals and Mining Act of 2007	The law vests the Head of State of Nigeria with power to make regulations for the prevention of pollution of any watercourse
3	The Public Health Act of 1917	It prohibits the fouling of water and vitiation of the atmosphere
4	The oil in Navigable Waters Act, 1968	It prohibits water pollution by oil spillage
5	The Petroleum Act, 1990	It covers prevention of pollution by inland waters, rivers, lakes and watercourses.
6	The River Basin Development (RBDA) Decree 25 of 1976 (repealed by No.87 of 1979 and also latter by the RBDA Act, Decree 35 of 1987,i.e.Cap 396)	In its present form Cap 396 spells out diverse functions and objectives for these Authorities to ensure a Pan-Nigerian program for water resources development.

7	The Environmental Impact Assessment (EIA) Decree, No.86 of 1992	The law seeks to protect the physical and aquatic environment.
8	Water Resources Decree, No.101 of 1993)	It vests the right to use and control all surface waters and groundwater and of all water in any water course affecting more than one state in the federal government, with provisions that any person may take water without charge for his domestic or livestock watering purposes (in any watercourse to which the public has free access)
9	The 1999 Constitution of the Federal Republic of Nigeria	The constitution puts in the Exclusive Legislative List (ELL) shipping and navigation on the River Niger and on any of its affluent and on any such other inland waterway as may be designated by the National Assembly to be an international waterway or to be an interstate waterway. The ELL also includes water from such sources as may be declared by the National Assembly to be sources affecting more than one state
10	National Policy on Environment 1989	Protection of the environment
11	National Guidelines and standards for Environmental pollution control in Nigeria (1991)	Pollution control in watercourses as part of the environment
12	National Effluent Limitation Regulation 1991	Control of discharge of industrial waste and sewage into watercourses
13	Pollution Abatement in Industries and Facilities Generating wastes Regulation 1991	Control of industrial pollution
14	Waste Management Regulation, 1991	Waste Management

Source: Updated from Akpabio, 2010.

4. Water and Community in Nigeria: Perception, Relationship and Management

Water resource represents a common property resource in rural Nigeria with social, cultural and economic significance to the livelihoods of the people. Consequently, decisions about its management have often generated enormous interest most especially when such decisions touch on individual and collective rights. By Bromley's (1991) classification, rights to resources could be encapsulated under state property regime (government has exclusive right over the resource); or private property regime (resource right rests with individual or corporation); or common property regime (individuals lay claims on collective goods as members of organized group); or open access (no property regime with no secure claims). Biswas and Mukherjee (2011) have argued that water resource qualifies as a common resource given that it is accessible to a whole community or collectively owned or managed by identifiable community to which no individual has exclusive property right. Whichever property regime water resource falls, the central fact remains that a clear authority system is usually needed over the resource as a way of guaranteeing the security and use propriety. The need for such authority system arises because of the broader question of how appropriate to govern natural resources shared by many individuals and groups in common. Indeed the phrase 'the tragedy of the commons' is often equated with the degradation of the environment when many individuals use a scarce resource in common. Using a case of an open pasture, Hardin captured what he referred to as the 'tragedy of the commons' as follows: '...each man is locked into a system that compels him to increase his herd without limit-in a world that is limited. Ruin is the destination toward which all men rush, each pursuing his own best interest in a society that believes in the freedom of commons' (Hardin, 1968: 1, 244).There are other similar views around this. For instance numerous analyses in modern economics run in the consensus that where many users or group of users have access to a common-pool resource, the total of resource units extracted will certainly be higher than the optimal economic level withdrawn (Ostrom, 1990: 3, cited Clark, 1980 and Dasgupta and Heal, 1979). Robert Smith (1981: 465) had observed that 'it is by treating a resource as a common property that we become locked in its inexorable destruction. In the context of natural resource management in developing countries, Caruthers and Stoner (1981: 29) observed that without public control, 'overgrazing and soil erosion of communal pastures, or less fish at higher average cost' would result. This observation led them to conclude that 'common property resources require public control if economic efficiency is to result from their development (Ostrom, 1990: 9).

Despite the seeming consensus of the inevitability of 'the tragedy of the commons' in a common property, a growing number of scholars over the years have brought some evidence to the fact that 'commons property' could generate opportunity and incentives for collective action and rules (Ciriacy-Wantrup and Bishop, 1975; Ostrom, 1990; Knox et.al, 1998). Ciriacy-Wantrup and Bishop (1975) particularly disagreed with the 'tragedy of the commons' hypothesis of Hardin for its failure to account for the existence of numerous common property arrangements, and their potential for encouraging sustainable resource utilization. The 'tragedy of the commons' could even be applied to a property whose right or institutions are not well adapted to the local circumstance. Ostrom (1990: 214) seems to observe along this line with regard to a public property whose rules are not effectively crafted and appropriately enforced when she argued as follows: '...but the tendency to try to impose uniform rules throughout a jurisdiction, rather than specialized rules that apply to localities within a jurisdiction, makes it extremely difficult for public officials to set up and enforce rules that will seem effective and fair to local appropriators.'

One of the distinguishing characteristics of indigenous system of natural resources management in Nigeria is the overlap of various authorities and rights system. For example the water resources management systems in Akwa Ibom state, currently imply a dual right system derived from: (a) Unrecognized or informal community based property right to water; and (b) Recognized or formal state right to water. If there is any difficulty attempting to draw a distinguishing line between these rights system in the urban areas, such difficulties is even more pronounced within local resource users, as 'common property' concept defines their daily activities and interaction with resources. It is useful to state that various levels of authorities are involved in water management in Nigeria namely, the individuals, local, state and the federal governments (see Table 2).

Table 2: Rights to Water Resources Management in the CRB

Institutions	**Rights and Responsibilities**	**Remarks**
Private Individuals	Right to water resources is linked to land rights	Mostly groundwater
Local Governments	Restricted to water resources in the rural areas of their jurisdiction	Powers subject to state and federal control
State Governments	Restricted to water resources in the urban areas and local government headquarters within their jurisdiction	Powers subject to federal control
CRBDA	Manages water resources of the entire basin catchments comprising of the two states- Akwa Ibom and Cross River	Powers not exclusive and still subject to state cooperation and permit
Federal Ministry of Water Resources	Has the exclusive rights and authority over the water resources of the entire country	Delegates powers of administration to different departments, RBDAs and the NWRI within the ministry.

Source: Akpabio, 2010.

When the urban and rural areas are further compared, one still observes a marked dualism in the way water is managed between the two socio-economic spaces. While the formal rights system to water (human, property and contractual rights) are applicable and enforceable in the urban areas, the rural communities, on the other hand, see water in the spectacle of prevailing tradition and spirituality and this affect the way water resources are managed at the local level. In consequence, there has been, at the moment, a tripartite interest in water management. These include private interest (whose authority is derived from the land use Act); community interest (the informal authority); and government interest (at various levels) (see Figure 2).

Each of the interested parties uses various management means, including customary practices, technical and technological abilities, economic, legal, legislative and political powers as management, access or utilization tools. Local communities are more at home with the usual customary and spiritual view of water and so would want its management correspond with taboos, sacrifices and customs. Such relationship is founded on reciprocal principles whereby members collectively develop interests and rules that promote accountable use of water. Private individuals' access to water is legally and legislatively enhanced by the Land use Act, which opens opportunity for those with economic power, land ownership, and political connection to have unlimited access to water resources especially at urban areas. Governments (represented at federal, state and local levels), on the other hand, adopt direct legal, legislative and political instruments to access water for public development and use purposes in a lineal, and most often exploitative manner through endless 'politically motivated' supplies. These instruments, however, conflict with the peoples' spiritual and symbolic attachments with water resources especially where such government services are not relevant, leading to friction in management claims. Using the few cases of public water resources based projects in Akwa Ibom State, the paper argues that where appropriate community involvements in water resources management are not secured, State water resources-based projects in rural areas often become victims of 'inexorable exploitation' which eventually will lead to the breakdown of such projects.

Figure 2: Levels of Interest in Water Resources Utilization in Akwa Ibom State

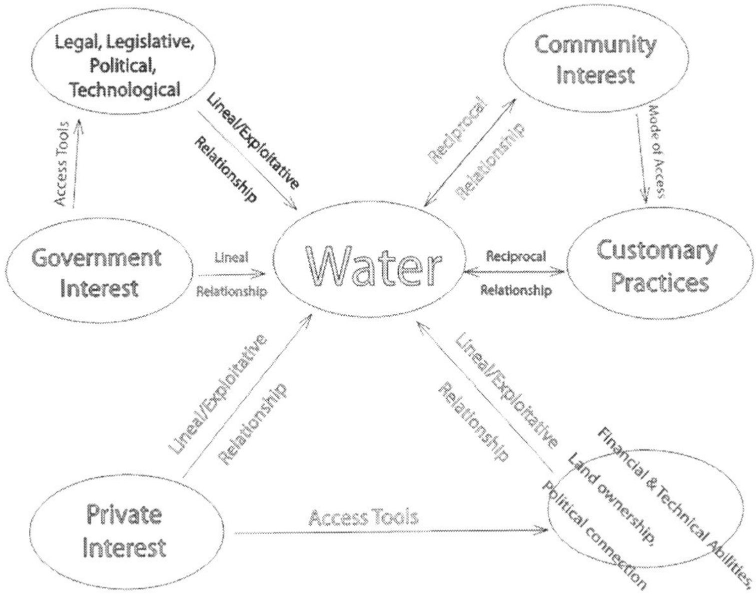

5. The CRBDA Water resources-based projects in local communities

The CRBDA runs a number of water resources-based projects including irrigation, dams and drinking water supplies in local communities in Akwa Ibom state. How do these projects fare, in the contexts of local cultural and social relations with water resources project communities? Two irrigation schemes namely, Abak and Itu were of particular interest because of recurring disagreements and tension that often characterize the smooth running of those schemes.

The Abak irrigation project was commissioned in 1991 and it covers an estimated area of 92.6 hectares, with two communities namely, *Abak Usung Idim* and *Abak Usung Atai*, claiming ownership of the affected land area. The Abak River provides the water source, which is adjacent to the project. Prior to 1991, the CRBDA had been involved in direct cropping alongside farmers with such crops as maize, cassava, cowpea, pineapple and vegetables. Actual channel and canal construction started in 1989 in preparation for irrigation farming. The project is jointly managed by the CRBDA and the village land allocation committee[1] especially in the allocation of farm plots to farmers and when need for irrigation arises. The land allocation committee works hand in hand with the management of the project in the allocation of farm plots as well as negotiating on behalf of farmers for irrigable water. For instance, the committee meets at every farming season to work out modalities for allocating plots to prospective farmers within the Basin Authority rate of N1000.00 (about $7.00) per plot per farming season.

The Itu irrigation project (located at Oku Iboku), on the other hand, is a multipurpose project incorporating irrigation, drainage and flood control. The site was initially a rice project, but it had been folded up for the irrigation and drainage project. The farmers are involved in horticultural practices with few plots leased out to individual farmers at a cost of ten thousand Naira (N10000.00) or seventy-six US Dollars (about $67.00) annually. Presently this project is not developed to the designed capacity and part of the problem for its underutilization has to do with the difficulties of having full access and control over the resource area because of unresolved questions bordering on ownership and control between the CRBDA and the local communities.

Nkari earth dam (located in Ini Local Government Area of Akwa Ibom State) is another classic case of contestation over resource ownership between public authorities and the local resource communities. Nkari is a clan, which comprises of 10 villages. The earth dam project was conceived in the 1960s as a multipurpose dam. It was then under the control of the Eastern Nigeria Development Corporation which later metamorphosed into the Cross River Basin Authority in the early 1970s.According to members of the communities, little compensation was paid at this time to the communities. Although the actual amounts could not be specified, it was gathered that whatever was paid had been used for community development (e.g. building of a community school).Prior to 2001 when the Federal Government decided to actualize its earth dam construction, individuals and the entire communities had been utilizing the land and available water resources in a variety of ways to improve their living condition. However, government plan to commence construction of the dam in 2001 consequently displaced the locals without any clear form of resettlement or compensation. The communities, however, used such government renewed interest in developing the place as bargains for pipe borne water supplies, electricity supply to all the communities; access roads to the affected rural communities as well as employment opportunities. However, as the project has not fully taken off, the realization of such expectations seems not possible. This has translated into persistent tension and sometimes outright violence given that so much local resources (in the forms of water and land) have been taken over by the CRBDA without commensurate compensation. The greater part of the tension has always been compounded by the suspicion of benefit capture by the privileged elites in the community, a situation which translates into persistent poverty for the greater majority.

The above cases illustrate how difficult to successfully run public water-based projects in local communities. Local media reports of vandalization of public drinking water schemes in local communities are quite common and almost on a weekly basis. Basically, common problems associated with public water resources-based projects in local communities could come as a result of outright rejection, reckless exploitation or vandalization of associated infrastructures. The root of such problems border mostly and fundamentally on local norms, beliefs and expectations. The first instance is the contradiction between the state modern water management norms which espouses cost recovery, commoditization and individualization on the one hand, and local belief in water as a 'free gift from nature', of which no cost should be imposed nor private right assigned, on the other hand. Take the Abak irrigation project for instance. While the native farmers may grudgingly pay for other services provided by the CRBDA (e.g., land preparation), this has not been the case with respect to any effort at recovering the cost of irrigation services. Given that native farmers are not also well-disposed to the participation of alien farmers (who could possibly enhance the prospect of cost recovery for irrigation services) the CRBDA is consequently constrained to running the services on almost full subsidization (see Table 3).

Table 3: Pricing/Cost Recovery and User Compliance in the CRB Projects

Pricing/cost recovery policy	Domestic water use	Irrigation	Industrial/ commercial	Power/ generation	Remarks
Full cost recovery	Nil	Nil	Not developed	Not developed	Projects run as social services. Domestic water use is free.
Partial cost recovery	Nil	Nil	Not developed	Not developed	Projects run as social services. Domestic water use is free.
Full subsidy	Yes	Yes	Not developed	Not developed	For irrigation, less than 1% of cost is charged on farmers to fuel pumping engine.

Source: Akpabio, 2010.

The prompt involvements of the village Chiefs and members of the communities though contribute in reducing the level of tension, can only achieve a short-lived result unless the fundamental cultural problems at the root of community disagreements with public projects are resolved.

Public acquisition of land and water resources create the fear of gradual dispossession of 'freely available' natural and 'God given' resources from the locals to be possessed by private individuals who have the means and resources to exploit them. Such growing tendency to impose commodity values on water in local communities implies placing the rich at a much privileged position over the poor, and this has serious equity implication in communities where the greater majority of the populace is very poor. Often times, such scenario is at the root of all reported cases of vandalization of public drinking water schemes with price tags. In general, wherever there exist conflicts between the public authorities and local communities over resource management, the consequence often come by way of enormous pressure on the contested resources; as in when governments developed water projects do not encourage best use. Such externally initiated projects (as in Itu and Abak) automatically confers some form of rights of free, reckless and 'revenge' use – 'revenge' in the sense of taking their portion of the 'national cake'. Even as government projects, the communities still perceive as common properties. More so, since there has not been any customary notion or general sense of involvement or inclusion in such project, its usage is even more reckless and cannot attract any 'protective' or accountable management as it would have been with a typical community owned resource project. Such negative perception is reinforced especially when such project is not a product of genuine community need. When a public property is perceived as a common property, the following characteristics apply among the users, namely:

1. Such a project is state initiated and funded project-in this case an opportunity to share in the 'national cake' syndrome. The 'share in the national cake syndrome' arises because of the prevalence of endemic corruption and ethnicity within the national, state and local polities.
2. One can waste it, mismanage or misuse it with reckless abandon;
3. Recovering cost of investments is absolutely impossible, which is linked to the 'national cake' syndrome;
4. Everybody competes to use it with no sense of accountability or responsibility;
5. Unwillingness to adhere to rules and regulations regarding use sometimes leading to vandalization;
6. Community norms are hardly brought to bear in utilization and management especially if 'needs' and 'interest' factors were not the major drivers of such public project.

These characteristics behaviors are compounded by ecological, religious, customary, economic and institutional factors. Ecologically, there is water abundance making it impossible for the affected communities to realize its value (Akpabio, 2005, 2006 and 2011). There is also the attitude of seeing water as 'a gift from nature' which implies free access and use to every member of the community irrespective of class or socio-economic status as opposed to outright commoditization or individualization which tend to limit access to those who can afford it. Looking at the economic perspectives, it could be argued that the impracticability of achieving cost recovery among the people is related to the massive poverty that has been the recurring nightmares of the rural populace in Nigeria (see Akpabio, 2004 and 2009). More so, Akpabio (2005) and Akpabio et.al (2007) having observed difficulties in cost recovery as the most common problem facing government water schemes in Nigeria attributed the problem as compounded by the absence of public trust in government services over the years especially when people see government projects as opportunity and their turn to have a share in the 'national cake'. The authors went on to substantiate this fact when they observed that people are very willing to pay for half a liter of water (in sachet form) at N10.00 than pay for a 25 liter of government water at N5.00. Taking example of the CRBDA projects, the above explanation has demonstrated the impossibilities of achieving cost recovery in project developments at every water use sectors. Even when domestic water use is free as a matter of policy, recovering costs for irrigation water becomes impossible and in most cases generate restiveness and conflicts among users.

6. Concluding Remarks: The challenges for state institutions

It is of interest to observe two forms of attitudes on water and public water projects especially among rural communities in Akwa Ibom state. The first is the spiritually loaded knowledge which defines and consolidates human-water relationship within the cultural contexts of the community. The second is the 'freebie' attitude to state water-based projects which tends to encourage their reckless use. The first perspective captures the social and cultural importance of water beyond its pure materialistic conceptualization espoused by the modern water resources management. Such modern management norms as commoditizing or individualizing water resources are conceptually and practically capable of marginalizing a large segment of social groups especially in the lower socio-economic class while at the same time privileging a very small segment of individuals in the upper socio-economic class. Packaging water resources-based project in a form that is little or not very sensitive to the human right and cultural imperatives of local communities places such a project at the risk of 'bungling' since the primary concern of the local majority revolves around long-term and future guarantee of their social and cultural rights to water in the emerging order of modern control. The context for which rural livelihoods are built in most developing countries especially in Africa depends on massive relationship with nature and natural resources as well as functional social capital rooted on culturally sanctioned norms. Compared to the urban dwellers, rural peoples' livelihoods are synonymous with poverty and weak government presence by way of physical and social infrastructures. Consequently, poverty itself offers remarkable leeway for the thriving influence of beliefs and traditional values whose contents and practices are diametrically opposed to modern system of natural resource management. On the other hand, modern system of managing natural resources derive from the western norms which tend to privilege humans above natural resources. Such contradictions are very fundamental and most often set the local communities against State agents when natural resource-based projects are to be established. As Vandana Shiva (2002) has rightly argued, the way water is conceptualized and represented is instrumental in determining who gains access to it and on what terms. This spontaneously could catalyze tension and conflicts over contestations of meanings and values given that the social power equations often weight significantly to the advantages and privileges of a select group bent on foisting a certain attitudes and orientation on the socially disadvantaged.

Reconciling these conflicting and dual but competing perception systems should be the first priority before water-resource based projects are set up. The practice of dialoguing and stakeholder meetings between government agents and prospective project communities will be practically helpful before any water-based resource project is conceived for development. Such a dialogue or meeting should be a regular component of a pre-and post-water resource-based projects development initiative as a way of giving voice, learning from the community perspectives and jointly devising means of addressing their concern. Akpabio et al. (2005) has found these participatory engagements very capable of promoting inclusion and a sense of ownership among project communities. Relevant government agencies also have a big role to play in the light of the lessons drawn from the above analyses. For instance Itu and Abak are not 'resource problems areas'. There is relative abundance of water, which may not elicit fullest interest on government projects from the communities examined. The more rational approach to handle such a situation by government agencies should have been based on demand responsive project targeting approach. Although the influence of ecological factors dictated the siting of such projects at the study areas, the study has shown that such assumption is not fruitful where traditional attitudes predominates, in addition to the non-appreciation of the 'scarcity value' of water by the affected communities. It would have been more fruitful and welcome by the people if such water resource-based projects were located in the northern parts of the Cross River Basin such as Ini and Ikono local government areas, which are confronted with relative scarcity as a result of their peculiar hydrological nature.

Notes

1 The land allocation committee is made up of two Chiefs and five members (each representing the two land donor communities) while the project officer is the chairman.

References

Akpabio, E. M. (2011), 'Water and people: perception and management practices in Akwa Ibom State, Nigeria', in *Society and Natural Resources*, 24(6): 584-596.

Akpabio, E. M. (2010), '*Integrated Water Resources Management in Nigeria: Local Factors and Institutional Challenges*, Germany: Lap Lambert Academic Publishing.

Akpabio, E. M. (2009), 'Indigenous Approach to Water Management in Nigeria: Making Sense of the Stigmatized Elements'. *Conference Proceedings: Endogenous Development as an Alternative to Africa's Development: Myths, Realities and Options for Poverty Reduction and Socio-economic Development*, The University for Development Studies, Tamale, Ghana October 27-30.

Akpabio, E.M. (2005), 'Assessing integrated water resources management in Nigeria: insights and lessons from irrigation projects of the Cross River basin', in *Water Policy*, 9(2): 149-168.

Akpabio, E. M. (2006), 'Notions of environment and environmental management in Akwa Ibom State, south-eastern Nigeria' in *Environmentalist*, 26: 227-236.

Akpabio, E.M (2004), '*The status of water supply and management in the cross-river basin, southeastern Nigeria*', Presented at an International Workshop on Water Resources Management for Local Development. Loskop Dam, South Africa, November 8-11.

Akpabio, E. M., Watson, N. M., Ite, U. E. and Ukpong, I. E. (2007), 'Integrated water resources management in the Cross River Basin, Nigeria', in *International Journal of Water Resources Development*, 23 (4): 691-708.

Akpabio, E. M., Imoh E. Ukpong; Nigel M. Watson and Uwem E. Ite (2005), 'Integrated water management and local institutional empowerment: a lost opportunity in the Cross River basin, Nigeria?' In G. N. Mathur and A. S. Chawla (Editors), *Proceedings of the XIIth World Water Congress,* 1: 297-309, New Delhi, India, 22-25, November.

AKS (1989), 'Physical Background, Soils and Land Use and Ecological Problems' *Technical Report of the Task Force on soils and Land Use Survey of Akwa Ibom State*, Uyo, Akwa Ibom State Government Printer.

Biswas, S. and Mukherjee, S. (2011), 'Understanding common property resources and environmental degradation in the vulnerable states of India-a Perspective', *IEMCON 2011,* Organised in collaboration with IEEE, India.

Bromley, D. W. (1991), '*Environment and economy: property rights and public policy'*, Oxford, UK: Blackwells.

Carruthers, I. and Stoner, R. (1981), 'Economic aspects and policy issues in groundwater development', *World Bank Staff Working Paper*, No. 496, Washington, D.C.

Clark, C. W. (1980), '*Restricted access to common property fishery resources: a game theoretic analysis*', In P. T. Liu (ed.): dynamic optimization and mathematical economics, New York: Plenum Press, pp.117-32.

Ciriacy-Wantrup, S. V. and Bishop, R.C. (1975), 'Common property as a concept in natural resources policy', in *Natural Resource Journal*, 15: 713-714.

Dasgupta, P. S. and Heal, G.M. (1979), *Economic theory and exhaustible resources*, Cambridge: Cambridge University Press.

Donahue, J. and Barbara, R. J. (1998), '*Water, culture and power: local struggle in global contexts*', Island Press, Washington, D.C.

Ekong, E. E. (2003), '*An introduction to rural sociology*', Uyo: Dove Educational Publishers.

Faniran, A. (1981), 'The human factor in the application of improved technology: the case of irrigation agriculture in water deficiency regions of the world', *4th AAASA*.

Groenfeldt, D. (1991). 'Building on Tradition: indigenous irrigation knowledge and sustainable development in Asia', in *Agriculture and Human Values*, 8(1-2): 114-120.

Hardin, G. (1968), 'The tragedy of the Commons', in *Science*, 162:1243-1248.

Knox, A., Meinzen-Dick, R. and Hazell, P. (1998), 'Property rights, collective action and technologies for natural resources management', SP-PRCA Working paper No. 1. IFPIR.

Kuruk, P. (undated), 'Customary water laws and practices: Nigeria', Available at: http://www.fao.org/Legal/advserv/FAOIUCNcs/Nigeria.pdf.

Linton, J. (2010), 'What is water? the history of a modern abstraction', University of British Columbia Press.

NPC (2007), *Census Reports*, National Population Commission, Nigeria.

Ostrom, E. (1990), '*Governing the commons, the evolution of institutions for collective action*', Cambridge University Press, New York.

Shiva, V. (2002), '*Water wars: privatization, pollution and profit*', South End Press. Cambridge, M. A: Canada.

Smith, R. (1981), 'Resolving the tragedy of the commons by creating private property rights in wildlife', in *CATO Journal,* 1(2): 439-468.

Sokile, C. S. and Van Koppen, B. (2004), 'Local water rights and local water user entities: the unsung heroines of water resource management in Tanzania', in *Physics and Chemistry of Earth,* 29: 1349 – 1356.

Acknowledgement

I thank the Alexander von Humboldt Stiftung for funding the expansion of this project whose initial conceptualization was facilitated by a small grant from the British Academy, London (VF2008/49121).

Chapter 5

Integrated Water Resources Management (IWRM) in South Africa –Challenges of Microbiology Quality of Water Resources

Rasheed A. Adeleke & Cornelius C. Bezuidenhout

1. Introduction

Water is an essential part of life. It is found and needed everywhere in the world. Water is characterized by special attributes that enable it to be constantly in motion, passing from one state to another, and from one location to another. Such characteristics of water have made water management a very difficult process (Biswas, 2004). Although water is everywhere, availability, quantity and quality of world's fresh water is limited and vulnerable (Radif, 1999; Biswas, 2004). Global water problems are constantly changing with time and differ significantly from one region to another, one season to another, as well as one year to another. Due to these complexities, solutions to water problems are therefore linked to many factors that include water availability, water management as well as competence and capacities of the institutions that manage them. Other factors include prevailing socio-political conditions that dictate water planning, development and management processes and practices, appropriateness and implementation statuses of the existing legal frameworks as well as availability of investment funds (Thomas and Durham, 2003; Biswas, 2004). Hence, in order to solve water problems, it is necessary to address issues about social and environmental conditions of the concerned countries as well as levels of available and usable technology. Furthermore, other equally important aspects of solutions to water problems include national, regional and international perceptions, modes of governance, educational and development conditions, and status, quality and relevance of research that are being conducted on the national, sub-national and local water problems (Thomas and Durham, 2003; Biswas, 2004). It is in this regard that the Integrated Water Resources Management (IWRM) has become a means of addressing the global water problems and working toward a sustainable future for water management (Xie, 2006).

2. Integrated Water Resources Management in South Africa

There are increasing numbers of governments throughout the world that are in the process of adopting or have adopted IWRM but majority of such countries are concentrated in the North (developed countries) (Moriarty, 2004). However, South Africa is a unique country of the South (developing country) where the National Water Act of 1998 was based upon IWRM principles and is in the long-term process of establishing new institutions at the catchment level to manage water resources (Moriarty, 2004). In the National Water Resource Strategy of 2004, IWRM was defined as "a process which promotes the co-ordinated development and management of water, land and related resources in order to maximise the resultant economic and social welfare in an equitable manner without compromising the sustainability of vital ecosystems". It is a management method that is intended to create harmony between the use of resources for livelihoods and conservation of the resource to sustain its functions for future generations, and promotes social equity, environmental sustainability and economic efficiency (DWAF, 2004).

As a semi-arid and developing country, South Africa needs to ensure extensive and efficient strategies and technologies are in place for sustainability of its water provision and management. With an estimated total loss from municipal reticulation systems of around 1 150 x106 m^3/a representing almost 30% of the system input of approximately 4 000 x106 m3/a. in 2005, there is still need for improvement (Seago and Mckenzie, 2007; Mckenzie and Wegelin, 2009). Therefore, considerable development is further needed in future especially in the areas of Water Demand Management (WDM) and supply side management. Such development will ensure appropriate improvement in time to support the ever growing demands for water in South Africa (Mckenzie and Wegelin, 2009).

The South African water acts (Act No 36, 1998) can be interpreted as the system that ensures human beings come first i.e. a basic water supply for human needs must be satisfied before water can be allocated for any other uses. The South African water policy reform highlights the primacy of social equity and basic human rights, which may take priority over ecological sustainability (Bohensky, 2009). The main focus of South African water policy ensures equity in order to address past issues of historical legacy of racially skewed land ownership as well as water accessibility/distribution (Moriarty, 2004). Further explanation of the South African water policy can be expressed in three ways. Firstly, through the use of ecological sustainable development principles where all activities are assessed according to the effect on river flows and assessed accordingly. Secondly, basins are grouped according to ecological classes from natural to critically modified and lastly, the need for restoration of unfair assignment of historical water interests, where legitimate claimants (black people) have been denied access due to past institutional or governance arrangements (DWAF, 2004; Bohensky, 2009).

In South Africa, the IWRM implementation is managed by Department of Water Affairs (DWA) through a catchment-based system that usually involves one or more local governments (DWAF, 2004). There are different examples of IWRM implementation in various catchment areas or cities in South Africa e.g. Mthata Catchment Forum, Kat river valley Catchment forum, Emfuleni Local Municipality etc. However, there have been reported problems for some water catchment areas in South Africa. These problems are usually associated with technical capability of DWA, inability of water managers to properly translate the written forms of IWRM concepts into practical forms and many institutional challenges that persist as a result insufficient alignment and cooperation between the policies of different government departments and the practices of different water sectors that impact on water (Funke et al., 2007).

3. Microbiological quality of South African water

The concern about South African water quality has been a subject of discussion in recent years. Both chemical and microbiological qualities of South African water have been questioned. A combination of inadequate or poorly functional water infrastructure services and the issue of communities' development poses serious economic and health implications for downstream users and this may subsequently affect the natural functioning of the river ecosystems (DWA, 2009). Other factors such as geology, geomorphology, soils, climate, vegetation, land use and land cover as well as pollution have been highlighted as major threats to South African waters (Pretorius, 1999; Hamilton-Attwell, 2007; van Niekerk et al., 2009).

Faecal pollution of water resources in South Africa has become one of the serious water problems in the country. This has been attributed to lack of appropriate sanitation infrastructure and poorly maintained wastewater treatment works in many parts of South Africa. As the custodian of South African water resources, the Department of Water Affairs (DWA) responded through the creation of the national Microbial water quality Programme (NMMP). The NMMP was established to address the increasing problems of faecal pollution, associated health risks of faecal pollution to users and absence of coherent information on South Africa's microbial water quality (Kuhn et al., 2000).

In the year 2000, DWA released a report on the proposed identification and prioritization of areas in South Africa with a potentially high health risk due to faecal pollution of surface waters. In this report, effort was made to create a prioritised list of areas, where a National Microbial Water Quality Monitoring programme (NMMP) could be established. According to this document, the goal of the programme was to provide information needed to assess and manage the potential health risks to water users that are related to faecal pollution of South Africa's water resources.

After the establishment of NMMP, many studies had discovered faecal pollution and contamination of different water resources in the country. In a study by Germs et al., (2004), an unacceptable levels of faecal and coliforms contamination of Chunies River – Limpopo was reported. This fact makes the water unsuitable for domestic uses. In a similar study conducted by Momba *et al.* (2006a), the disinfection practices of small rural systems of the Eastern Cape and their effects on drinking water they supply to the communities were investigated. The study covered 55 plants across five rural district Municipalities (Cacadu, Chris Hani, Amathola, Ukhahlamba and O.R. Tambo). The outcome showed that rural water treatment plants are failing to produce safe drinking water due to lack of necessary technical expertise by the operators and lack of communication between consultants, operators and municipal officials on technical issues relating to plant operations.

In another study on Mhlathuze River by Lin et al., (2004), high levels of antibiotic resistance enteric bacteria were isolated from the river. The result indicated that such highbacterial levels could be a reflection of both industrial and human activities on this river. It was therefore suggested that the determination of antibiotic susceptibility and resistance patterns of microbes isolated from water resources should become part of the microbial monitoring process. Such recommendation was shared by Momba et al., (2006b); in their study where investigation of treatment removal of microbial and chemical contaminants was carried out in four wastewater treatment plants that serve the Buffalo City (Dimbaza, East London) and Nkokonbe (Alice, Fort Beaufort) Municipal areas in the Eastern Cape Province of South Africa. In that study, it was discovered that the general microbiological quality of the effluents from all the plants was poor as there were indications of high levels of contaminations by *Salmonella*, *Shigella*, *Vibrio cholera* and *coliphages*. The study therefore highlighted the problem with the current disinfection practices and guidelines as insufficient.

Furthermore, Bezuidenhout et al. (2002) and Obi et al. (2002) separately reported high levels of faecal contamination in Mhlathuze river and different water sources in Venda regions respectively through the detection of elevated levels of coliforms. In these cases, the water sources were being consumed for domestic, agricultural and industrial purposes.

In terms of monitoring microbiological water quality in South Africa, this has been done through three tiers that include national, regional and local governments (van Niekerk, 2004). However, according to Haigh et al., (2010), South African constitution has indicated that municipalities have the ultimate responsibilities for the delivery of water service and sanitation to consumers. In this regard, these roles include provision of safe potable water, sanitation, treating wastewater and effluent, effecting repairs together with preventative and major maintenance as well as revenue collection and related financial management. Having realised the enormous problems associated with the quality of South African water, the DWA introduced two different certification programmes; the Blue drop and the Green drop.

4. The Blue drop and the Green drop certification programmes

The Blue drop certification programme was initiated in 2005 and it is meant to assess the drinking water quality of South Africa. In this programme, both microbiological and chemical qualities of drinking water are used to award scores to different municipalities/regions of the country. From the recent report released for 2010, the average national Blue drop score increased from 53% in 2009 to 70.74% in 2010. With 55% of all municipalities scoring more than 50%, the outcome looks promising. However, there are still serious concerns about the 24% of municipal drinking water quality management programmes that are not up to standard. On the other hand, the Green drop certification process was established in 2008 to ensure compliance of waste water treatment methods. According to the 2009 report, South Africa has a large number of wastewater management facilities, which is made up of 850 municipal treatment plants, extensive pipe networks and pump stations. This has made the maintenance of the wastewater treatment facilities as well as the Green drop certification process more complex than that of drinking water facilities/Blue drop certification process. An illustration of this fact will be the City of Cape Town where the whole Cape Peninsula drinking water comes from just one water supply system. This same area is being served by 23 wastewater treatment systems. Outcome of the 2009 Green drop report indicated more than half of South African wastewater treatment facilities scored below 50%, a poor one indeed. Although outcomes of the Green drop assessments indicated that none of the facilities assessed was at a point of collapse, there are serious concerns over inadequacy of facilities, skills shortages at all levels, overstretching of facilities, poor understanding of technicalities of wastewater treatment as well as underfunding of facilities (DWA, 2009; DWA, 2010).

5. Conclusion

Quality and quantity of water are of great global importance in water management. There are great disparities in terms of water availability from one region to another due to many different factors. Factors such as seasonal variation and inter-annual variation have been highlighted to have very important impact on water availability (UN-Water, 2008). However, most developed countries have designed artificial method to deal with the natural problems associated with water availability. Such mitigating approach has ensured the reduction in potential risks to humans and environment that could be associated to water variability. Perhaps, the most important threat to water quality is pollution (UN-Water, 2008). Unfortunately, water pollution and poverty have been linked in many instances. While it is understandable that IWRM cannot solve all poverty problems, it is also important to know that no good strategy for poverty eradication can be successful except it is linked to strategies of water management. As mentioned in the NWRM document, provision of basic water and sanitation services is an important element of water's impacts on poverty eradication as it involves issues of health and hygiene as well as the processes involved in gathering and transporting water from remote, usually polluted sources (DWA, 2004).

The transformation of South Africa from apartheid to democratic governance has also reflected in the country's water policies. There is no doubt that South African water policies need constant review to accommodate increasing number of people as well as other developmental changes associated with economic improvements. There is definitely an urgent need to re-evaluate the IWRM practices in South Africa. It is necessary to establish, improve and update communication methods among all stakeholders in the country's water sector.

It is true that continuous investigation of pollution in all water bodies could be expensive; however, there are many solutions to such challenges. Development of a detection system that is handy, cheap and readily available will go a long way in solving water quality problems in South Africa. This can be used to test all water samples in the country from time to time. Wherever and whenever there is an indication of high levels of dangerous microbial contamination, further investigation in forms of studies can then be conducted. This makes more economic sense than the continuous investigations on water quality. In addition, diversity studies will also become very beneficial; this means knowledge of the microbial diversity can also be used indirectly to predict levels of pollution.

Lack of appropriate coordination of different researches being carried out in recent years on South African water resources is a clear indication of improper implementation of IWRM practices. Many authors (Obi et al., 2002; Bezuidenhout et al., 2002; Germs, etal., 2004; Momba et al., 2006a) have published outcomes of their researches indicating some potential dangers of South African water resources but did not mention how their discovery relates to NMMP or fit into the framework of IWRM practices in the country. It is clear that the microbial quality of South Africa water problems cannot be solved in isolation; it requires an integrated approach where all stakeholders will have roles to play. Although it is a good thing that many scientific research are been carried out on South Africa water resources, proper harmonisation of the outcomes of such studies into the framework of NMMP and IWRM practices in South Africa will make them more useful and more meaningful. As pointed out by Nomquphu, (2005), the proposed creation of a governance institution by DWA to coordinate and share resources, infrastructure, data and information among all stakeholders will be a good start to ensure that a straight-forward and uniform approach is endorsed by all role players.

References

Bezuidenhout, C. C., Mthembu, N., Puckree, T. and Lin, J. (2002), 'Microbiological evaluation of the Mhlathuze River, Kwazulu-Natal (RSA)', in*Water SA*, 28(3): 281-286.

Biswas, A. K. (2004), 'Integrated water resources management: a reassessment', in *Water International*, 29(2): 248-256.

Bohensky, E., Connell, D. and Taylor, B. (2009), '*Experiences with integrated river basin management, international and Murray Darling basin: Lessons for Northern Australia* (Chapter 22). Northern Australia Land and Water Science Review, full report.

Department of Water Affairs (DWA), (2009), 'Green drop report: South African waste water quality management performance', Department of Water Affairs, South Africa.

Department of Water Affairs (DWA), (2010), 'Blue drop report: South African drinking water quality management performance', Department of Water Affairs, South Africa.

Department of Water Affairs and Forestry (DWAF), (2004), *National Water Resource Strategy,* First Edition, , Pretoria, South Africa.

Funke, N., Oelofse, S. H., Hattingh, J., Ashton, P. J. and Turton, A. R. (2007), 'IWRM in developing countries: Lessons from the Mhlatuze catchment in South Africa', in *Physics and Chemistry of the Earth*, 32: 1237-1245.

Germs, W., Coetzee, M.S., van Rensburg, L and Maboeta, M.S. (2004), 'A preliminary assessment of the chemical and microbial water quality of the Chunies River – Limpopo', in *Water SA*, 30(2): 267-272.

Haigh, E. H., Fox, H. E. and Davies-Coleman, H. D. (2010), 'Framework for local government to implement integrated water re-

Chapter 6

Green Drop Certification of Wastewater Treatment Plants in South Africa –

An Initiative to Reduce Drinking Water Sources Pollution and Bedrock of Wastewater Reuse

James R Adewumi & Olawale O. Olanrewaju

1. Introduction

The growing community concerns about environmental pollution resulting from the quality of wastewater disposed into sensitive environments and diminishing freshwater source has become a popular topic of discussions among water professionals in South Africa. Since the available WWTWs are spread across the country, it is difficult to estimate the magnitude of the pollution problems resulting from indiscriminate disposal of wastewater. However, it is clear that streams and rivers in the Western Cape, Eastern Cape, KwaZulu-Natal and the Vaal have major problems with Total Dissolved Solids (TDS), and most of South Africa's rivers have eutrophication problems (NSER, 2007). Recently, Dzwairo and Otieno (2010) developed a tool that models variability of surface raw water quality to predict the cost of treating raw water to the required potable quality using Upper and Middle Vaal Water Management Area of South Africa as a case study. The paper concluded that the downstream water boards paid a higher water resources management charges for more polluted raw water than upstream water boards.

The quality of discharges from wastewater treatment plants into river and streams in South Africa is currently receiving the required priority attention as a matter of national importance. The National Water Services Regulation Strategy (DWAF, 2008) provides a clear statement of strategic intent to regulate the water and sanitation services sector in South Africa. The driving force of this strategy is the mitigation of risk associated with the management of water and sanitation facilities and the development of more comprehensive and effective regulation for the country. The three main programmes identified to mitigate risks are (DWAF, 2008):

- concentrated regulatory efforts to address compliance and performance problems in priority municipalities, particularly where risks pose threats to health and the environment;
- a national drinking water quality regulatory initiative to manage potentially serious risks associated with unsafe drinking water (Blue Drop Certification); and
- a national wastewater discharge regulation initiative to manage potentially serious risks to health and the environment (Green Drop Certification).

This paper focuses on the effort of the Department of Water and Environmental Affairs (DWEA) in implementing the third objective of the National Services Regulatory Strategy to regulate water and sanitation services and its implications in wastewater reuse in water scarce area of South Africa.

In fulfilling the stated third objective and in line with international good practice of wastewater management, DWEA embarked on the assessment of all wastewater treatment plants in South Africa in 2008 (Manus and van der Merwe-Botha, 2010). This assessment is aimed at developing the following two-pronged regulatory approach to raise the performance of wastewater treatment plants and effluent quality:

- an approach that is based on a risk profile of all wastewater treatment plants and that targets the plants that have the greatest impacts on the receiving environment;
- an incentive-based approach that recognises excellence in the wastewater industry. This is to encourage service providers (i.e. municipalities) to work towards the achievement of Green Drop Certification which acknowledges the state of excellence in wastewater services. A Purple Drop Certification is issued if a service provider fails to comply with a predetermined level of green drop.

The above two-pronged approach to wastewater treatment plant assessment allows for incentive, punitive or assisted measures to be taken depending on the specific circumstances of non-compliance by the wastewater management authorities. Communities in which their WWTW has been awarded Green Drop status can use this status to market their communities to both its citizens and tourists. Also, a Green Drop status will allow citizens to have a trusted information that wastewater is being managed in a sustainable and environmentally-acceptable manner. This information will better enhance the community acceptability of wastewater reuse in a water scarce area of South Africa like the City of Cape Town (CoCT).

2. Research Methodology

First order assessment and blue drop certificate initiatives

First Order Assessment and Green Drop Certification of municipal wastewater treatment works are government initiative through DWEA as the first step in multi-barrier system of ensuring safe drinking water quality. While First Order Assessment is geared towards information gathering to classify wastewater treatment works in terms of its potential to have high risks, Green Drop Certification process is an incentive measure of DWEA to municipalities with excellent wastewater treatment works performance. This initiative is aimed at solving the problems of non-compliance of municipal wastewater treatment service providers with the South African Water Acts. This process is driven by strengthening the regulatory approach whilst at the same time refocusing the Local Government in a manner that is more responsive to regulatory imperatives (DWEA, 2009).

A national roll out of both the First Order Assessment and the Green Drop process from August 2008 to September, 2009 campaigned successfully to channel the consumer's voice to raise political awareness. It is also aimed at bringing out positive changes to wastewater treatment and to set out the platform for more efficient planning and investment in wastewater services facilities and skills (DWEA, 2010).

The First Order Assessment provides a scientific and verifiable status of municipal wastewater treatment plants that will reveal any risk associated with a plant. This form the basis of regulatory intervention by prioritizing the higher risk plants and applying the Enforcement Protocol for Organ of State (a business process geared at solution formulation and rectifying non compliance situations). The risk rating of each plant within a municipality is calculated using cumulative risk rating (CRR) express as follows:

$$CRR = WF_1 \times (WF_2 + WF_3 + WF_4) \quad \text{.......................................1}$$

Where WF are weighting factors assigned to four high risks areas:
WF_1 = Design capacity of plant also represent hydraulic loading onto receiving water body
WF_2 = Flow amount exceeding, on and below capacity
WF_3 = Number of non-compliance trend (i.e. effluent compliance as discharged to receiving water body)

WF_4 = Compliance/non compliance (i.e. technical skills – supervisory, process control and maintenance)

$$CRR = \frac{CRR_{expected}}{CRR_{obtained}} \quad \ldots\ldots\ldots 2$$

The Green Drop Assessment is based on the scoring criteria listed in Table 1

Table 1: Green drop record card scoring criteria (DWEA, 2010)

<table>
<tr><th>Criteria</th><th>Score</th><th>Symbol</th><th>Description</th><th>Requirements (& Weighting)</th></tr>
<tr><td rowspan="7">Adequacy of process control, maintenance and management skill</td><td>100% (10)</td><td>A</td><td>Fully complies with all requirements.</td><td rowspan="7">Treatment works complying with Reg. 2834 of water Act., in terms of Classification and Registration. (20%).

Process controllers are complying with skills requirements of Reg. 2834 of Water Act. (50%).

Availability of skilled maintenance skills. (10%).

Operation and maintenance manual is in place. (20%).</td></tr>
<tr><td>80%-90% (8-9)</td><td>B</td><td>Complies with all requirements except 1.</td></tr>
<tr><td>70% (7)</td><td>C</td><td>Not complying with 2 requirements.</td></tr>
<tr><td>50% (5)</td><td>D</td><td>Not complying with criteria No. 2 or complying with No. 2 and none other.</td></tr>
<tr><td>30% (3-4)</td><td>E</td><td>Not complying with criteria No 1 & 2 or No. 2 & 4.</td></tr>
<tr><td>10%-20% (1-2)</td><td>F</td><td>Not complying with the majority of the requirements.</td></tr>
<tr><td>0% (and lack of information</td><td>G</td><td>Not complying with any of the requirements or the complete lack of information.</td></tr>
</table>

Criteria	Score	Symbol	Description	Requirements (& Weighting)
Efficient of wastewater Quality Monitoring Programme	100%(10)	A	Fully complies with all requirements.	Details of an effective Operation Monitoring Programme. Details of an effective Compliance Monitoring Programme. Proof of sufficient samples and determinants taken from sample sites.
	70%(7)	B	Complying with all requirements except 1.	
	60%(6)	C	Not complying with requirement No. 2 and another requirement. Or not complying with any other 3 requirement.	
	30%(3)	E	Only complying with 1 requirement. (1 or 2).	
	15%(1.5)	F	Not complying with majority of the criteria. Only complying with 1 requirement.	
	0%(and lack of information)	G	Not complying with any one of the requirements or complete lack of information.	
Credibility of Drinking Water Sample Analysis	100%(10)	A	Fully complies with all requirements.	Proof to be provided of the laboratory used. Laboratory is either accredited or participates in accredited proficiency scheme (obtaining an acceptable z-score). Proof that analysis results are used to improve process controlling.
	70%(7)	B	Complying with all requirements except for requirement No. 1.	
	60%(6)	C	Complying with all requirements except for requirement No. 3	
	30%(3)	E	Not complying with requirement No. 2 or not complying with requirements No. 1 & 2.	
	15%(1.5)	F	Only complying with requirement No. 3	
	0%(and lack of information)	G	Not complying with any one of the requirements or complete lack of information.	
Regular submission of wastewater quality results to DWA	100%(12/12months)	A	Fully complied with criterion	Results must be submitted by12th month of the year
	0%(<10months)	G	Less than 12 sets of data submitted to DWA. No data submitted.	

Criteria	Score	Symbol	Description	Requirements (& Weighting)
Wastewater compliance with license conditions/ General authorizations or special limits.	100%(35)	A	Fully complied with criteria.	Proof of wastewater quality compliance data for the past 12 months and copy of standards used. Provide figures per determinants; number of analysis per determinants & the number of non complying analysis per determinants. % compliance per determinant (measured against overall compliance %).
	80%(28)	C	Complies with most criteria except 1.	
	60%(21)	D	Does not comply with criteria 1 & 2.	
	20%(7)	E	Does not comply with criteria 3	
	0% (0)	G	Did not comply with both sub- criteria or failed to submit sufficient data for assessment purposes.	
Wastewater quality failure response management	100%(20)	A	Fully comply with criteria.	Proof of a documented effluent quality incident management protocol (or protocol similar in function) specifying roles and responsibilities. Provide evidence of implementation.
	605(12)	C	Have evidence to proof incident management control, but has no documented protocol.	
	40%(8)	E	Has a documented protocol in place but not evidence to proof implementation.	
	0% (0)	G	Not complying with criteria or failed to submit sufficient information for assessment purposes.	
Wastewater treatment capacity	100%(5)	A	Fully complies with criteria.	
	80%(4)	B	Complies with all criteria except one.	
	60%(3)	C	Not complying with 1 criterion.	
	40%(2)	E	Not complying with 2 criteria or criterion 2.	
	20%(1)	F	Only complying with one criterion	
	0%(0)	G	Not complying with criteria or failed to submit sufficient information for assessment purposes.	

The information and data used in assessing WWTWs were obtained from DWEA provincial offices, DWEA national electronic information systems, Water Service Authorities, Water Services Providers, Laboratories, and Consultants.

Data obtained from the above mentioned sources are: Municipal background and relevant information pertaining to wastewater services; Plant location, coordinates, owner and operator; Plant design capacity and receiving flows; License status; Effluent quality and permitted limit/standard (i.e. pH, Chemical Oxygen Demand, Electrical Conductivity, ammonia, nitrate and nitrite, ortho-phosphate, Suspended Solids, E. Coli and Faecal coliforms). Others are technical skills compared to Regulation 2834 requirements (i.e. supervisor, process controller, maintenance crew) (DWAF, 2004); Occupational health and safety appointments compared to legal requirements.

3. Results and Discussion

Table 2 presents the summary of the results of the cumulative risk rating (CRR) obtained from each province. It includes the number of wastewater treatment works per province and their CRR. This presents an overall risk profile of all plants in the country, which values were subsequently prioritised from highest to lowest order CRR values. According to the evaluation equation (equation 1), the lowest CRR that can be achieved is 1 (No risks) and the highest is 48 (Very high risky).

Table 2: Summary of the cumulative risk rating values in WWTWs in South Africa (DWEA, 2010)

CRR*	Eastern Cape	Northern Cape	Western Cape	Gauteng	KZN	Free State	Limpopo	Mpuma-langa	North West	South Africa
28						1			3	4
27	1		1							2
26										0
25			1	1						2
24				1	1					2
23	1			1	3	4			5	14
22		1	1	3	2				1	8
21	2		1	2		2				7
20	2		8	3	1	2				16
19		1	1	2	1	2			2	9
18	16	5	7	1	1	17	23	2	24	96
17	16	8	3	5	1	5	1	6	2	47
16	11	14	8	2	8	4	3	3	5	58

CRR*	Eastern Cape	Northern Cape	Western Cape	Gauteng	KZN	Free State	Limpopo	Mpuma-langa	North West	South Africa
15	10	13	15	3	6	8	2	6	1	64
14	9	5	10	2	15	14	6	7	5	73
13	16	7	21	3	7	12	7	6	2	81
12	10	7	11	5	9	15	5	13	1	76
11	15	4	15	2	17	5	8	11	1	78
10	9	3	12	5	12	2	5	11	1	60
9	4	2	10	5	20	2	1	5	3	52
8	2		14	2	12	1	1	5		37
7	1		10	3	14	2		3	3	36
6		1	6	1	10			1	1	20
5			1	1	5	1		1		9
4					1					1
Total WWTWs	**125**	**70**	**156**	**51**	**147**	**101**	**62**	**80**	**60**	**852**

**Cumulative risk rating; the red line indicates a possible target benchmark*

All the WWTWs that falls above the red line (CRR > 18) is an indication of high risks profiles WWTWs that needs first level of intervention to lower their constituted risks to drinking water sources and the environment at provincial level. The First Order Assessment indicated that none of the WWTWs assessed approached the highest possible risk value of 48. This implies that despite the high risks rating (CRR of 18–28), none of the WWTWs is at the state of total collapse. However, their adequate maintenance to meet the set criteria will reduce drinking water source pollution and provide a solid foundation for alternative source of water for non potable purposes through reuse. In general term, about 45% of the assessed WWTWs scored better that 50% against the stringent criteria set. However, the remaining 55% that scored between 0% and 49% require drastic steps to improve their operating conditions.

Most of the assessed WWTWs fail the First Order Assessment and were denied Green Drop certification as a result of at least one or combinations of the following reasons (DWEA, 2010):

- Manpower shortages at all levels of operations (i.e. from managerial to junior level). The result is that many WWTWs are not operated correctly and the resultant effluent water quality does not meet effluent disposal standards;
- A poor understanding of the technicalities of WWTWs is prevalent among senior management and administration officers. Therefore, the needs of the plant and its operation are denied the priority required;

- Lack of good understanding of the funding requirements for WWTWs operations by the senior management. This is further exacerbated by the additional burden placed on operators by municipal procurement procedures and its custodians-financial support for dealing with urgent issues at plants is, in many cases, non-existent;
- In many cases, the processes employed at WWTWs are no longer sufficient and often obsolete to deliver the required final water quality; and
- Many municipalities had no information on the wastewater treatment works they are responsible for. This gives room for a situation where no attempt is made to monitor effluent compliance.

Despite the above listed weakness in the assessed WWTS, of particular interest is that, out of 169 Water Service Authorities (WSA) assessed; only 7 WSA in 7 municipalities out of 262 municipalities in South Africa obtained Green Drop Certificates in 32 WWTWs they are managing. Detail of the municipalities and wastewater service areas are shown in Table 3.

Table 3: Green Drop Award in 2009 (DWEA, 2010)

S/Nº	Water Service Authority and Providers	Wastewater Service Area
1	City of Cape Town; Western Cape	Cape Flats
		Liandudn
		Macassar
		Melkbostrand
		Mitchells Plain
		Oude Kraal
		Parow
2	City of Johannesburg and Joburg Water; Gauteng	Bushkoppies
		Driefontein
		Ennerdale
		Goudkoppies
		Northern Works
		Olifantshoek
3	City of Tshwane; Gauteng	Daspoort
		Zeekoegat
4	Ekurhuleni Metro & ERWAT; Gauteng	Dekema
5	Ethekweni Metro, KwaZulu Natal (KZN)	Amazimtoti
		Central
		Craigieburn
		Phoenix
		Southern Works
		Umdloti
		Umhlanga
		Umhlatuzana
		Umkhomaas
		Umlazi
		Verulam
6	George Municipality; Western Cape	Kleinkrantz
		Outeniqua
7	Mbombela Local Municipality & Silulumanzi, Mpumananga	Kanyamazane
		Matsulu

In the face of continuous pollution of drinking water sources by indiscriminate disposal of poorly treated wastewater into rivers and streams with the fast diminishing of freshwater sources in South Africa, wastewater reuse present a sustainable unconventional source of non-potable water. Treated wastewater is a preferred unconventional water source, since the supply is increasing because of population and industrial growth. Reuse of treated wastewater will help in maintaining environmental quality and at the same time, relieve the unrelenting pressure on conventional, natural freshwater sources. While the nutrients in wastewater can assist plant growth when reused for irrigation, wastewater disposal, in extreme cases, is detrimental to the ecosystems of the receiving drinking surface water.

The Plus Economics Ltd (2010) conducted an economic impact

analysis of the impending water crisis in South Africa on various key macroeconomic. The analysis used two scenarios: a decrease in the quality of water provided in South Africa, and a decrease in the quantity. The analysis involves an annual, aggregate, structural dynamic macro-econometric model, as well as a static input-output model. The preliminary report identifies eutrophication of surface waters; heavy metal contamination; acid mine drainage; increases in salinity; increased levels of suspended solids; bacterial and viral pathogens; contamination by pesticides and organic pollutants as a major water quality risks. These problems can be largely traced to inadequate wastewater treatment and disposal to surface waters. The report further indicated that the effects of the tested scenarios are extremely alarming. Key macroeconomic variables, such as economic growth and disposable income per capita, are expected to contract due to the effects of poor water quality on total factor productivity. The effects on the individual economic sectors' gross operating surpluses and employment are also of great concern.

Water quality is a fundamental component of any economy, and diminishing quality will directly impact the economy through myriad channels, for example, food supply, which will in turn hamper labour productivity and poverty alleviation, as well as health and life expectancy. Also, the ability to produce, manufacture and provide services will be constricted. It was clear from the simulation results of Plus Economic Ltd (2010) that the water crisis scenario has a permanent impact on South Africa economy.

Effect of green drop certification on wastewater reuse in South Africa

With the records of successful wastewater reuse implementation in many developed and developing countries (Adewumi, *et al.*, 2010) and the new DWEA initiative of *Green DropCertification* of WWTWs discussed above, it has become imperative to evaluate the potential of wastewater reuse as a viable alternative in the drive towards overcoming the challenges of current and future water shortages in South Africa. Although there has been limited uptake of this alternative in many communities within South Africa, a few reuse schemes have been identified and discussed below.

Urban waste water reuse in South Africa is found in the Ethekweni Metro, the KwaZulu-Natal Province and the CoCT, the Western Cape Province. These two municipalities have the highest numbers of wastewater treatment works with Green Drop Certificate for 11 and 7 WWTWs respectively.

In the KwaZulu-Natal Province, a Public-Private Partnership exists between the Ethekweni Metro and private investors in the production of treated wastewater for industrial applications. The WWTWs is designed to treat 47.5 Ml/d of domestic and industrial wastewater with about 74% of the treated wastewater supplied to MONDI Paper[1] The treated wastewater produced meets or exceeds the South African drinking water standards (DWAF, 2004) in 95% of the parameters measured. Significant benefits of this project have included:

- delayed capital investment for increased marine outfall pipeline;
- delayed capital investment for future bulk potable water supply infrastructure;
- creation of long-term revenue from a levy raised on the production of recycled water;
- reduced cost of water services to Durban's citizens; and
- a 44% reduction in the 2001 water bill for MONDI Paper.

In the Western Cape Province, the CoCT stands out as one of the very few local authorities in South Africa that has operated a wastewater reuse system for several decades. Reuse has therefore become a vital component of the city's integrated water management plan. Treated wastewater is supplied from participating WWTWs to several large scale irrigation and industrial users. Wastewater reuse in the CoCT is grouped as follows (Adewumi *et al.*, 2010):

- Formal (direct) users of wastewater: this group of users are connected to a treated wastewater pipe network of 2527km from seven WWTWs. The pipe network is funded and operated by the local authority (Table 4).

- Private (direct) users of wastewater: these are users who privately fund and operate the treated wastewater pipe networks from the participating WWTWs (e.g. Century City and Steenberg golf estate from the Cape Flats WWTWs). These schemes withdraw approximately 14.5 Ml/d of treated wastewater.
- Informal (indirect) users of wastewater: a significant number of these users are unregulated and withdraw treated wastewater from downstream points along a surface water source after discharge from the participating WWTWs. These include some golf courses from the Athlone treatment works and agricultural users from Kraaifontein and Scottsdene (Table 5).
- Groundwater recharge: in Atlantis, drinking water is supplied primarily from the Atlantis aquifer with extensive recharge occurring using treated domestic wastewater. Two large infiltration basins, covering an area of approximately 500,000m² exist some 500m upstream of the drinking water extraction point. These basins recharge to the order of about 200 Ml/a (Murray et al., 2007).

Table 4: Formal wastewater reuse within the City of Cape Town (CoCT, 2007)

Wastewater treatment works	Volume of treated wastewater reused (Ml/d)	Reuse activities (%)		
		Sport field/ landscape irrigation	Industries	Agriculture
Bellville	4.10	28	71	
Kraaifontein	2.10	100		
Macassar	2.00	100		
Parow	1.50	100		
Potsdam	27.60	9	48	43
Scottsdene	0.70	100		
Wesfleur (Atlantis)	0.30	100		
Total	**39.90**			

The CoCT supplies treated wastewater to only large non-domestic consumers. Public safety and costs of retrofitting are the major reasons why domestic consumers are not allowed access to the effluent. The introduction of Green Drop Certification of wastewater treatment plants will provide public with trusted information on treated wastewater and boost public acceptance of reuse.

Table 5: Informal wastewater reuse within the City of Cape Town (CoCT, 2007)

Wastewater treatment works	Volume of wastewater reused (Ml/d)	Reuse activities (%)		
		Sport field/ landscape irrigation	Industries	Agriculture
Athlone	3.00	100	-	-
Borcherds Quarry	2.00	100	-	-
Cape Flats	4.60	100	-	-
Gordonsbay	0.50	100	-	-
Kraaifontein	5.50	-	-	100
Melkobs Strands	2.00	100	-	-
Potsdam	2.40	100	-	-
Scottsdene	5.00		-	100
Total	**25.00**			

Adewumi *et al.* (2010) reported that significant potential for wastewater reuse by large non-domestic consumers for non-drinking applications still exist in CoCT. However, trust on the service providers to produce safe effluent that will not compromise public health is a prerequisite to public acceptance of wastewater reuse. Perception surveys conducted by Po *et al.* (2004) showed that trust in the Water Corporation of Western Australia to provide safe and reliable treated wastewater was critical to why residents were willing to reuse wastewater. Questionnaire administered to the CoCT treated effluent consumers shows that trust in the service provider to supply the appropriate quality of treated wastewater was 48%. This response is poor and likely influenced by the poor qualities of treated wastewater that have been supplied these respondents over time prompting further on-site treatment of the effluent before use by many consumers (Adewumi *et al.*, 2010). With the introduction of Green Drop Certification of WWTWs in South Africa, it is obvious that the level of acceptance of treated wastewater reuse will drastically increased over time.

4. Conclusion

With the introduction of Green Drop Certification of wastewater treatment plants in South Africa, the Department of Water and Environment Affairs has taken a bold step to safeguard the treated effluent receiving rivers and streams which also double as the source of drinking water. This initiative could be best regarded as the first step in multi-barrier system of ensuring safe drinking water quality. If the current assessment on WWTWs can be continued and sustained, then the problems of non-compliance with effluent disposal quality by the municipal wastewater treatment service providers will be reduced if not totally eliminated. This paper present the results of the first assessment of wastewater treatment plants in South Africa and the implication on wastewater reuse in water scarce area of South Africa. Many WWTWs failed to meet the requirements for the award of Green Drop Certificate because of the poor management style and ageing infrastructure. In water scarce area of South Africa where treated wastewater is being reused for non-potable purposes, consumers trust on service providers will be better enhanced with Green Drop Certification while at the same time, the receiving rivers and streams will be better protected.

Notes

1 Integrated packaging and business paper producing company

References

Adewumi, J. R., Ilemobade, A. A. and van Zyl, J. E. (2010), 'Treated wastewater effluent reuse in South Africa: Overview, potential and challenges', in *Resource, Conservation & Recycling* 55(2): 221-231.

CoCT, City of Cape Town (2007), 'Treated effluent re-uses strategy and master planning within the City of Cape Town', *BVi Consulting Engineers- BVi Report,* No. C1500/1.1, April..

DWAF, Department of Water Affairs and Forestry (2004), 'Revision of General Authorizations in terms of section 39 of the National Water Act 1998 (Act No. 36 of 1998) - engaging in a controlled activity', *Government Gazette* 26187, Pretoria.

DWAF, Department of Water Affairs and Forestry (2008), 'National

Water Service Regulation Strategy: Protecting the interest of the consumer and public through the effective regulation of water supply and sanitation services'. Available at: http://www.participation.org.za/docs/natwater.doc

DWEA, Department of Water and Environment Affairs (2009), 'Green drop Report 2009 version 1: South African wastewater quality management performance'. Available at: http://www.pmg.org.za/files/docs/100429 GreenDropReport.pdf.

DWEA, Department of Water and Environment Affairs (2010), 'Wastewater treatment works list'. Available at: http://www.dwaf.gov.za.

Dzwairo, B. and Otieno, F. A. O. (2010), 'Integrating quality and cost of surface raw water: Upper and Middle Vaal Water Management Areas South Africa', in *Water Science & Technology: Water Supply*, 10 (2): 201-207.

Manus, L. and van der Merwe-Botha, M. (2010), 'Raising wastewater treatment performance through incentive and risk-based targeted regulation', in *Proceedings, Water Institute of South Africa* (WISA), Durban, South Africa 18-22 April.

Murray R., Tredoux G., Ravenscroft P. and Botha F. (2007), 'Artificial recharge strategy', *Water Research Commission Report*, Pretoria. ISBN 1-86845-450-9.

NSER, National State of Environmental (2007), 'Report on freshwater systems and resources'. Available at: http://www.environment.gov.za/soer/nsoer/issues/water/pressure.htm#climate.

Po M, Kaercher, J, and Nancarrow, B. (2004), 'Literature review of factors influencing public perceptions of water reuse', Melbourne: CSIRO Land and Water.

Plus Economics (Pty) Ltd (2010), 'The South African water crisis: an economic impact study', Available at: http://www.polity.org.za/article/the-south-african-water-crisis-an-economic-impact-study-november-2010-2010-11-16.

Chapter 7

Impact of Climate Change on Water Resources in Africa

Oghenerobor B. Akpor & Maxwell K. Boakye

1. Introduction

There is a general awareness in Africa that a large number of the population in different areas are currently suffering adequate and efficient water supply and distribution. Despite this awareness, spatial and temporal detailed information on freshwater availability and scarcity is still lacking (Schuol et al., 2008). Although the Africa continent with a land area of nearly 300 million square kilometres holds a wealth of natural resources (minerals, forests, wildlife and rich biological diversity), which only a few parts of the rest of the world can match, the continent also has some of the driest desserts, largest tropical rain forests, highest equatorial mountains in the world, with most of the key resources highly unevenly distributed (Urama and Ozor, 2010).

The availability of fresh water is a vital vulnerable resource in any country. Water is a key resource for the sustenance of life and society through agricultural production, industry, and hydro power, as well as health and human development at large (Shakespear,

2007). Continents such as Africa, where adaptation mechanisms are weak or uncoordinated, are especially vulnerable to insecurity related to water, food, energy, and natural disasters. This will be a major challenge not only for African countries but also international partners involved in climate change mitigation and adaptation efforts. In Africa development, water quality and quantity issues seem to pose significant burdens to sustainable development (Access, 2009). Because of rapidly growing urban populations, with average growth rates of 5% per year, reports have shown that by 2025, in addition to the existing water stressed countries, 12 more countries will be classified as water scarce. When this occurs, the number of individuals without clean water access will increase from 100 million to 400 million. This will pose a great and growing challenge to sustainable development (Garrity, 2005; UNEP, 2010).

According to the United Nations Development Programme (UNDP), the over a decade achievement in human development is likely to be slowed down or reversed because of climate change. This is because of emerging and continuous threats to water and food security, agricultural production and access, nutrition and public health. This has led to prediction of 600 million people being pushed into malnutrition and an increase of 1.8 million people facing water scarcity by 2080, if the current impacts of climate persists (UNDP, 2008; Ludi, 2009). A warmer earth is expected to lead to many projected changes in the coming decades. Some of the changes include: widespread drought and flooding, sea level rise and retreating glacier. Africa as a continent has experienced some of these changes already, especially rainfall patterns and rise in sea levels, and it is projected that there is a most likely experience in greater intensity in the future (Osman-Elasha, 2009).

Analyses of models on climate have revealed that the number of people who are at risk because of water scarcity increases with increasing temperatures towards the second half of the 21st century. The impacts of such scarcity are suggested to be much larger in arid and semi-arid regions than what global averages suggest (Urama and Ozor, 2010). Because, no community and economy will prevail without water of sufficient quality and quantity, the security implications of climate change are of increasing relevance to international peace and security (Access, 2009). In most African countries, shortages and stress of fresh water are posing serious threats to economic growth, social cohesion and political stability. Several countries in Africa are already experiencing huge water stress due to the effect of insufficient and unreliable rainfall and changing rainfall patterns and flooding. The current Africa estimate revealed that water stress is being experienced by 25% of the population (about 200 million people), with more countries expected to face future risks (Ludi, 2009). Also, the increase in the scale of severity and impact of climate change is suggested to likely exceed the coping capacity of many communities and countries. When this happens, it could lead to severe socio-economic and environmental problems; hence will require more effective adaptation efforts than what it is at present (Osman-Elasha, 2009). This paper was therefore aimed at reviewing current impacts of climate change on Africa water resources. Based on current literature, Africa vulnerability and adaptation to climate change were also discussed.

2. Climate Change Effects on Africa's Water Sources

Although Africa is the least responsible continent for climate change, with Sub-Saharan Africa producing less than 4 per cent of this waste – known as "greenhouse gases" – far less than North America, Europe, Asia and other industrialized regions, it is the most vulnerable to its effects. Because Africa is regarded as the most vulnerable to climate variability, a situation aggravated by the interaction of multiple stresses that occur at varying levels and low adaptive capacity. Various economic sectors are already vulnerable to current climate sensitivity, with huge economic impacts. Some of the effects include reduction in agricultural productivity, worsening in food security, and change in frequency and distribution of rainfall, thus leading to increasing incidences of floods and droughts. Others include, spread of diseases and increasing risk of conflict over scarce land and water resources, with the long term impacts of climate change, which will include change in rainfall patterns, which will have effect on agriculture, reduce food security, economic growth and other challenging hurdles in meeting the Millennium Development Goals

(MDGs). Generally, the major areas of concern with respect to climate change are water resources, agriculture, health, ecosystems, biodiversity, forestry and coastal zones. Based on the experiences in different African countries, some of these effects are summarised in Table 1 (Ali-Dinar, 2007; APF, 2007; Urama and Ozor, 2010).

Historically, Africa climate change record shows an approximate 0.7°C warming over most of the twelfth century. There is also a decrease in rainfall over large parts of the Sahel and an increase in rainfall in East Central Africa. In the next century, it is predicated that global warming trends will lead to changes in the pattern of precipitation, rise in sea level and increased frequency of other extreme conditions (Desanker, 2010). Summarily, with an assumed rapid growth in economy and a balance in energy resources, it is hypothesized that in the next 100 years, the following will be observed:

- Warmer drier subtropical regions than the moister tropics
- A much hotter and drier (up to 4°C or more) Northern and Southern Africa with a fall in precipitation up to 15% or more.
- Likely adverse effects on wheat and maize production in the North and South, respectively
- Increase in average rainfall in eastern Africa, including the Horn of Africa and parts of Central Africa.
- Increase in the spread and severity of vector-borne disease e.g. malaria.
- Rise in sea levels by up to half a meter in the next fifty years, thus causing serious consequences in parts of West Africa and the Nile Delta (Conway, 2009).

3. Climate change and flooding in Africa

A large portion of Africa is susceptible to flood, with reports showing that it is the most prevalent disaster in North Africa, the second most common in east, South and Central Africa and the third most common in West Africa (Urama and Ozor, 2010). In major parts of Sub-Saharan Africa, extensive floodplains and wetlands are in existence. Despite serving as critical contributions to the livelihoods of many people, these ecosystems depend on frequent flooding. Since these ecosystems are utilised extensively for agriculture and fishing activities, the loss of these ecosystems will also have a more direct effect on local populations, hence their long-term preservation and sustainable use is critical for economic and social well being of current and future generations (Rebelo and Finlayson, 2010). In Africa, flood-related fatalities are reported to have increased over the years. This increase in flood intensity is attributed to the effect of global warming and the growth in population, human activity and developmental patterns, thus leading to increased human vulnerability to the impacts of climate change (2011).

According to a BBC News report of 17th September, 2007, more than a million people across a swathe of 17 African countries were reported to be suffering from the effects of severe floods. The report revealed that as a result of the aftermath of the flood a total of 250 died and hundreds of thousands of homes were washed away on some of the continent's most fertile land, with the UN fearing the floods could lead to major outbreaks of water-borne diseases such as cholera and dysentery. The brunt of that flood was felt more in Uganda, Ethiopia and Sudan in Eastern Africa and in Ghana, Burkina Faso, Togo, Mali and Niger in Western Africa. The majority of these countries and others were said to be facing yearly outbreaks of floods, thus prompting some governments to set up contingency plans (BBC, 2007).

Also, in a CNN report of 8th September, 2009, torrential rains and flooding were reported to have affected 600,000 people in 16 West African nations. The worst hit countries were Burkina Faso, Senegal, Ghana and Niger with 159 human deaths at the time of the report. In addition, roads and buildings were ruined from Mauritania to Niger. In Agadez, Niger, a town about 458 miles (738 km) north of the capital, Niamey, close to 988 acres (400 hectares) of vegetable crops and hundreds of livestock were reported to have been washed away. The report also revealed that in 2007, 300 human deaths and 800,000 people due to the aftermaths of floods (CNN, 2009).

Table 1: Climate change related effects on water resources in Africa

Regions	Climate change related effects
Central Africa	Hot, dry dusty harmattan winds affecting northern areas Floods, droughts and landslides are common Volcanic activity with periodic releases of poisonous gases from Lake Nyos and Lake Monoun
East Africa	Frequent and recurring droughts and dust storms in summer months and floods in rainy seasons Geologically active Great Rift valley, susceptible to earthquakes and volcanic eruptions
North Africa	Mountainous areas subject to severe earthquakes, mudslides and floods in rainy season Hot, dry dust-laden winds lasting one to four days in springs and fall, dust storms and sand storms Northern mountains that are geologically unstable and subject to earth quakes Periodic droughts, flash floods, landslides, hot and dry windstorms occurring in springs
Southern Africa	Periodic droughts, seasonal August winds blowing from the west, carrying sand and dust, which can obscure visibility Local heavy rainfall, causing periodic flooding in the plateau Prolonged and recurring droughts, floods, tropical storms and cyclones
West Africa	Dry sand-laden harmattan winds blowing from the Sahara, which is common in dry seasons (December to February) Periodic and recurring droughts and floods Hot harmattan wind, which can reduce visibility Significant drop in rainfall in some parts e.g Gambia, where rainfall has dropped by 30% in the last 30 years

Source: Adapted and modified from Urama and Ozor, 2010.

In another report, flood is said to have displaced about 2.5 million people in Africa in 2009 and more than a million in 2007. Overall, the report revealed that from 1950 to 2009, African flood fatalities is said to have increased by a factor of 10, with over 15, 000 people dying during the decade 2000-2009 (Schewe, 2010). Although the report has claimed upswing in flood deaths in Africa over the past decades is due mainly to human settlement pattern, rather than a consequence of climate change, the overall impact of climate change in the increased flood pattern cannot be ignored. In August 2009, unusually heavy rains lasting six hours were reported to have deluged the city of Khartoum in Sudan. Although higher wealthier parts of the city were reported not to have been relatively affected, the vast shanty towns that surround the city centre were largely affected, with report of 27 deaths and over 20,000 homes damaged and destroyed (Geospace, 2010).

The above-mentioned incidences of floods in Africa are not in isolation. Fourteen countries in Africa, namely Burkina Faso, Chad, Ethiopia, Ghana, Kenya, Liberia, Mali, Niger, Nigeria, Senegal, Sudan, Togo, Uganda and Rwanda are reported to be worst hit by flood in recent years (Urama and Ozor, 2010). From a number that was fewer than 2000 in 1950 to 1969; flood-related deaths increased to more than 15,000, between 1990 and 2009. Apart from the number of deaths, the number and extent of negative impacts on life and the economy is also reported to have increased substantially. Although several arguments and views are reflected by different individuals, the most obvious factor behind this trend is a reflection of climate-driven rise in the intensity of precipitation and flood magnitude.

4. Climate change and drought in Africa

Drought is a sustained and regionally extensive occurrence of below average natural water availability. There are four major forms of drought conditions: meteorological, agricultural, hydrological and socio-economic droughts. During meteorological drought, atmospheric conditions results in deficiencies of precipitation change from one area to another. In the case of agricultural drought, which affects food production and farming, precipitation shortages bring about soil water deficits, reduced ground water or reservoir levels, and so on. Hydrological drought associated with the effects of periods of precipitation shortages on water supply. When this drought occurs, water in hydrologic storage systems, such as reservoirs and rivers are often used for multiple purposes such as flood control, irrigation, recreation, navigation, hydropower, and wildlife habitat.

On the other hand, socioeconomic drought occurs when the demand for an economic good exceeds supply as a result of a weather-related shortfall in water supply. This is because the supply of many economic goods, such as water, forage, food grains, fish, and hydroelectric power, depends on climatic conditions (Gommes, 1996; Urama and Ozor, 2010).

Although it is difficult to discriminate from other human influences, over the last decade, numerous studies have been published about climate change and drought-related issues. The African continent has a long history of rainfall fluctuations of varying lengths and intensities, with the worst droughts being those of the 1910s, which affected East and West Africa alike, which were generally followed by increasing rainfall amounts, but negative trends where observed again from 1950 onwards culminating, in West Africa, in 1984. Since then, starting in 1988, the Sahel has recorded a series of good (Gommes, 1996). However, in recent years, several cases of severe droughts within the continent have been reported in recent years. In 2007, between January and March, hot, dry weather that wilted crops was experienced in southern Africa. According to the report, the severe drought produced near-record temperatures that combined with rainfall, caused extensive crop damage. Because farmers could not plant in the dry conditions and many of the crops that were planted wilted in the dry heat, the impact was a drop in anticipated corn crop from ten million tons in December to six million tons in April. The last reported drought of that magnitude in South Africa was reported to have occurred in 1992 (NASA, 2007).

Over the last 20 years, there have been increased frequencies of drought in Eastern Africa with projections that it is likely to continue as long as global temperatures continue to rise. This will pose increased risk to the estimated 17.5 million people in the Great Horn of Africa who currently face potential food shortages. Because global temperatures are predicted to continue to rise, it is anticipated that average precipitation totals in Kenya and Ethiopia will continue to decrease or remain below the historical average. "The decreased rainfall in Eastern Africa is most pronounced in the March to June season, when substantial rainfall usually occurs, thus leading to food shortages" (ScienceDaily, 2011). According to a news report, drought was reported to have left more than eight million people in East Africa short of food and water, and the number could rise sharply if funding to help them is not increased. The report indicated that, if appropriate action was not taken immediately, the current drought had the potential to be as devastating as that of 2009 in which over 20 million people in Kenya, Somalia, Ethiopia, Uganda and Eritrea faced life-threatening food and water shortages following consecutive years of failed rains (News24, 2011). Also, in 2010, severe drought that affected over 10 million people was reported to cause increased hunger across four countries in West Africa. In Niger, which was the worst-affected country, 7.1 million were reported to be hungry, with nearly half considered highly food insecure because of the loss of livestock and crops coupled with a surge in prices. In Chad, two million people were reported to require food aid while the eastern parts of Mali and northern Cameroon were also badly affected by the failed rains (Environment, 2010).

5. Climate change and water availability/quality in Africa

Across Africa, because of great disparity in water resources, a quarter of all people are experiencing water stress (between 1000 and 1500 m^3 per capita per year). In most African countries, due to increasing population, water scarcity (less than 1,000 m^3 per capita per year) is presenting a major development challenge. It is reported that in 1995, water scarcity was experienced in 10 African countries (Algeria, Burundi, Cape Verde, Djibouti, Egypt, Kenya, Libya, Malawi, Rwanda and Tunisia). Recent projections have indicated that by 2025, the situation is expected to be worsened, with 14 countries expected to suffer water scarcity and 11 suffering water stress. It is further projected that if the current water demand situation persists, all sub-Saharan African countries will fall below the level of having sufficient water for their population and a majority of them being in a state of either water-stress or scarcity (Syngenta, 2010). Some predictions on the impact of climate change on water availability in Africa revealed that warm sea surface temperatures may lead to increased droughts in equatorial and subtropical areas. Also, with less precipitation during already dry months, there is the likelihood of increased desertification and complete disappearance of the Kimanjaro's glaciers by 2015-2020 (WWF, 2006).

Globally, observation in recent decades have revealed climate-related warming of oceans, lakes, rivers and other water bodies, with implications for fresh water ecosystems, such as alterations in water salinity, water nutrient content, concentration of pollutants, water chemistry and pH balance (Urama and Ozor, 2010). Because of changing climatic conditions, a lot of African rivers are reported to have experienced flow decrease. For example, in the Nile region, most scenarios of water availability have estimated a decrease of more than 75 % in river flow by the year 2100. At higher temperatures and lower flows, there is a widespread decrease in water quality. For example, the presence of sediments, nutrients, dissolved organic carbon, microbial pathogens and pesticides will increase due to higher water temperatures, more intense rain and longer periods of low flow. When this happens, there will be an increase in risks to human health, increase in cost of water treatment and negative impacts on water ecosystems (Nyong, 2005; CSIR, 2010). The presence of elevated concentrations of naturally occurring elements in water, such as arsenic, fluoride, etc, can have catastrophic health impacts (MacDonald, 2005).

6. Vulnerability and Adaptation to Climate Change in Africa

Africa is a continent where the effects of climate change are being most hardly felt. In Africa, the effects of climate change, such as rising temperature and changes in precipitation are undeniably clear with impacts already affecting ecosystems, biodiversity and people, with future impacts predicted to worsen. The vulnerability of Africa is due to the lack of economic, development and institutional capacity (WWF, 2006). Several research reports have consistently reported on the vulnerability of the continent to the impacts of climate change. This vulnerability is attributed to the combination of physical and social factors, which represent the interface between climate threat exposure and other non-climatic threats, and the capacity to cope with them (Nyong, 2005). Because most African countries are dependent on natural resources and the agricultural sector for food, employment, income, tax revenue and exports, changes in weather conditions could have great impacts on incomes and livelihoods. Besides, poor countries and communities are most likely to have their assets and wealth tied up in natural resources; hence damage to the natural resource base is most likely to be more damaging to these counties. At present, a third of Africa's productive land is classified as dry land and with climate change tending to bring less rainfall and shorter growing seasons, such dry lands may extend further. With little irrigation in Africa and most farmers practicing subsistence farming, there is much reliance on rainfall, thus there is high degree of vulnerability to even slight changes in rainfall patterns. Finally, with weak governments and institutions in most African countries, coupled with the brain drain of qualified people to the developed countries, so many people will have to cope on their own (Conway, 2009; Ernie, 2011).

Given the fact that the impacts of climate change are enormous, both short and long-term adaptation response strategies are vital. There is the need for such responses to be anticipatory, rapid, empowering and enabling to individuals and communities at various levels. Although a broader and more comprehensive adaptation effort that focuses on three measures that target the interface between poverty and vulnerability is advocated, most adaptation efforts in Africa are based on the four dimensions (income and material needs, health and basic education, rights and empowerment, and social-cultural affiliation and security) of poverty/basic needs (WWF, 2006; Eriksen et al. 2008). According to Eriksen et al. (2008), a comprehensive adaptation must entail the following measures:

- Targeting the risk posed by climate change to poverty, which may include provision efficient social infrastructures, viability of cropping system and other sources of livelihood.
- Strengthening coping and adaptation capacity to climate stress e.g. engagement in alternative sources of income during drought, accessing forest products and seasonal movement of livestock for grazing
- Addressing the causes of vulnerability, such as poor market re-

lations in trading in niche drought products or poor health facilities and the spread of infectious diseases such as HIV/AIDS and ensuring the labour capacity of household.

According to Schulze, 2010, South Africa faces four key issues in climate change research and adaptation. In his report he outlined the issues as the need to mainstream climate change challenges into coordinated national strategies and action plans, and the formalisation of a climate change adaptation strategy, which is more specific to the water sector. Furthermore he stated the need for researchers to address in vigour second and third order impacts of climate change on the water sector (e.g. impacts of extremes, variability, groundwater recharge, dynamics of projected changes in land use interwoven with effects of climate change, consequences of changes in water quality, terrestrial and aquatic ecological responses, conflicts over shared international waters and vulnerability of the poor). A final identified need is that of addressing climate change on complex operational catchments, i.e. those that are already largely water engineered instead of natural hydrological systems. These issues and many more can be extended to the majority of African countries as a whole.

Since climate change is capable of hindering the achievement of the millennium development goals, combating it is vital for the pursuance of sustainable development. It is argued that adaptation to climate change is an inevitably complex process as the phenomenon of climate change itself. This is because in designing appropriate countermeasures that are both cost effective and socio-politically acceptable, each of the impacts requires proper assessment. Any meaningful response to climate change must involve both mitigation (controlling greenhouse gases to stabilise climate change to an acceptable limit) and adaptation, which entails adjusting to climate change impacts given the existing levels of greenhouse gases in the atmosphere (Nyong, 2005; Conway, 2009). Also, to promote and guide sustainable resource management, the provision of clear and comprehensive structures is fundamental. This will require legal and institutional frameworks that are reboust and unambiguously stipulates the main principles and strategies that need to be adhered to for conservation and sustainability of natural resources such as water

(Urama and Ozor, 2010).

Although the Sahel have been known to be long vulnerable to drought, thus leading to improvement and food insecurity, its experience in recent decades reveals what adaptation to climate change may mean in reality. While the people in the Sahel have adapted to climate change, the process has not been cost free. Consistent drought due to decease in rainfall since the 1960s have made livestock to be herded further south, away from the desert margins into settled, cultivated areas where accommodation between animals and crops is sought. As a result of this, although herders succeeded in finding their livestock tracks and grazing areas ploughed up, farmers were faced with the challenge of stopping hungry animals from straying into fields and gardens in search for pasture. As a coping and adaptive technique, farmers have shifted to shorter-cycle varieties of millets and maize while avoiding crops that need higher rainfall. Others have resorted to digging wells and building small dams to provide sufficient water for the cultivation of economic crops like onions, tomatoes, etc (Trech et al. 2007).

In Cameroon, rainfall is reported to have declined by 2% per decade since the 1960. With changing and unpredictable rainfall patterns, "Green Care", a local NGO based in Cameroon has been running tree planting workshops with communities in the highlands. The aim of the project is to ensure the restoration of native forest around village catchments, which will in turn protect water supplies. Although the project is reported to have faced series of serious challenges, since 2007, a total of 11,718 trees have been planted, with 98% of them reported to be indigenous. The replanted tree cover will act as stores for rain when it falls and the water is released more slowly than where there is no tree cover, thus regulating water flows from springs and stream heads. When this happens, more water is stored in the soil since the speed of runoff is reduced and water is allowed to soak into the soil. Also, in Uganda, because of changing rainfall patterns, severe droughts have occurred in most parts of the country in recent years, especially in the northern and western parts, thus leading to food insecurity and social conflicts. To cope, farmers have either resulted to alternative farming types that require less water or adapted other coping measures (Osman-Elasha, 2009).

A major challenge to the design and implementation of specific adaptation strategies to climate change in most African countries is the uncertainty of the impacts of climate change. It is therefore argued that adaptation strategy that will be both meaningful and efficient should ensure that efforts are made to become independent of stable and/or regular climate patterns, such as extension of irrigation facilities, where applicable. At present, although the majority of climate models are able to reproduce observed African climate in its general patterns (overall trends, large-scale spatial patterns), they most often display deviations on a more detailed level. In addition, concrete efforts should also be made for the diversification of income structures that will lead to societal flexibility in responding to changing environmental conditions (Muller, 2009). In addition, for effective adaptation strategies, it is suggested that a framework of adaptive management, supported by more-local economic analysis and stronger orientations is vital for adaptation of Africa's water sector to changing climatic conditions (UNEP, 2010). Furthermore, because of the imbalance in the state of water resources in increasing urbanising Africa societies, the calibration of water demand with available supply is a vital step in reducing climate change effects. This will however require effective sector-wide policies and institutional reforms that will help to improve water demand management and services coupled with associated environmental health gains. A viable institutional reform is expected to improve organisation capacity, which can help to secure sustainable public and private water and wastewater investment, regulation of providers in a more effective way, demand management and effective water supply management that could help arbitrate water allocation during drought conditions (Shakespeare, 2007).

7. Conclusion

This paper has described climate change impacts on water resources, with specific focus on floods, droughts and water availability and quality in Africa. The paper also discussed Africa vulnerability and adaptation approaches to climate change. It is obvious that the effects of climate change, such as changes in floods and drought patterns, poor water quality and decrease in surface and groundwater

water availability are real, with impacts already affecting people, ecosystems and biodiversities. It is argued that both human and natural activities, (evaporation, transpiration, flow regimes, ground water table and sea level) have effects on all sections of the hydrological cycle. Despite the fact that no conclusive evidence is yet to be available to substantiate the cause and effect relationship of climate change and water resources, given the current African vulnerability level and its effects on the economy and food security, it is obvious that the negative impacts will be greatest in Africa. This situation is aggravated by the interaction of multiple stresses occurring at various levels and low adaptive capacity.

Due to existing developmental challenges, although there is a high degree of uncertainty on the impacts of climate change on African societies and ecosystems, there is agreement that climate will change, even more strongly than the current global average. Since the present and future consequences are too risky to ignore, adequate mitigation and adaptation steps are vital to protect Africa water resources. Given the present degree of vulnerability, any workable and efficient adaptation step will need concrete support by all stakeholders and must be viewed as a continuous process which will address the present climate variability and future climate risks.

References

Access (2009), 'Climate change and security in Africa', in *Africa Climate Change, Environment and Security Dialogue, Vulnerability Discussion Paper*. Available at: http://www.gcca.eu/usr/ClimateChangeSecurity _Africa_VulnerabiltyDiscussionPaper.pdf.

Ali-Dinar, A.B. (2007), 'Africa: climate change impact report', *Africa Focus Bulletin,* Dec. 2. Available at: http://www.africafocus.org/docs07/cc0712b.php.

APF (2007), 'Climate change and Africa', 8th *Meeting of the Africa partnership Forum*, Berlin, Germany, 22-23 May.

BBC (2007),'Millions hit by flood in Africa', *BBC World News Online*. Available at: http://news.bbc.co.uk/2/hi/6998651.stm.

CNN (2009), 'West Africa flooding affects 600,000, U.N. reports',

CNN World Online. Available at: http://articles.cnn.com/2009-09-08/world/west.africa.flooding_1_burkina-faso-wfp-flooding?_s=PM:WORLD.

Conway, G. (2009), 'The science of climate change in Africa: impacts and adaptation', *Grantham Institute for Climate Change DiscussionPaper No 1*.

CSIR (2010), 'Water resources', *Council for Industrial and Scientific Research (CSIR) Climate Change Studies*: K2C.

Desanker, P.V. (2010), 'Impact of climate change on life in Africa', *WWF Climate Change Program Report*.

Environment (2010), 'Severe drought causes hunger for 10 million in West Africa'. Available at: http://www.guardian.co.uk/environment/2010/jun/03/drought-hunger-west-africa.

Eriksen, S., O'Brien, K. and Rosentrater, L. (2008), 'Climate change in Eastern and Southern Africa: impacts, vulnerability and adaptation', in *Global Environmental Change and Human Security Report* 2.

Ernie, T. (2011). 'Flood fatalities in Africa linked to settlement patterns', in *Eos, Transactions American Geophysical Union,* 92(1): 12-24.

Garrity, D., Malesu, M., Khaka, E., Mati, B., De Bock, T., Nyabenge, M., Odour, V. and Odour, A. (2005), 'Potential for rainwater harvesting in Africa: a GIS overview', in *Final Draft Report, United Nations Environment (UNEP) and RELMA, Draft Report*.

Geospace, (2010), 'Population trends, not climate, causing increased flood fatalities in Africa'. Available at: https://blogs.agu.org/geospace/2010/10/15/population-floods-africa.

Gommes, R. (1996), 'Rainfall variability and drought in Sub-Saharan Africa', in *Sustainable Development, Food and agricultural Organisation of the United Nations, Discussion Paper*.

Ludi, E. (2009), 'Climate change, water and food security', in *Overseas Development Institute (ODI) Background Note*. Available at: http://www.odi.org.uk/resources/download/3148. pdf.

MacDonald, A.M. (2005), *Developing groundwater- a guide for ru-*

ral water supply, ITDG Publishing.

Muller, C. (2009), 'Climate change impacts in sub-Saharan Africa? an overview and analysis of scenarios and models', in *German Developmental Institute Discussion Paper 3*.

NASA (2007), 'Drought in Southern Africa'. Available at: http://earth observatory.nasa.gov/ NaturalHazards/view.php?id=18226.

News24 (2011), 'Drought worsens East Africa hunger', *News24 online*. Available at: http://www.news24.com/Africa/News/ Drought-worsens-East-Africa-hunger-20110427.

Nyong, A. (2005), 'Key vulnerabilities to climate change in Africa: global warming', in *Looking Beyond Kyoto Conference*, 21-22 October, Yale Centre for the Study of Globalisation.

Osman-Elasha, B. (2009), 'Adapting to climate change in Africa: managing Africa's water in a changing climate', in *Jotoafrika*, Issue 2.

Rebelo, L. and Finlayson, M. (2010), 'Characterisation of inland wetlands in Africa', in *International Water Management Institute K&C Science Report* – Phase 1.

Schewe, P.F. (2010), 'Fatal floods in Africa: human settlement patterns, not climate change, are responsible for an increase in deaths', in *Inside Science News Service*, Dec 15.

Schulz, R.E. (2010), 'Climate change and the South African water sector: where from? where now? where to in future?'. Available at: http://www.dwaf.gov.za/aww/vdfileload /file.asp?val=22& tablename= Event Session Docs2&fld=ID.

Schuol, J., Abbaspour, K.C., Yang, H., Srinivasan, R . and Zehnder, A.J.B. (2008), 'Modelling blue and green water availability in Africa', in *Water Resources*, 44: 1-18.

ScienceDaily, (2011), 'More frequent drought likely in Eastern Africa', in *ScienceDaily online*. Available at: http://www.sciencedaily.com/releases/2011/01/110128113426.htm.

Shakespeare, W. (2007), 'Climate change adaptation in the water sector in the Middle East and North Africa: a review of main issues'. Available at: http://www.fao.org/fileadmin/user_upload/

rome2007/docs/Climate_Change_Adaptation_Water_Sector_NENA.pdf.

Syngenta (2010), 'Africa's water quality: a chemical science perspective', in *SA Report by the Pan African Chemistry Network.*

Trench, P., Rowley, J., Diarra, M., Sano, F. and Keita, B. (2007), 'Beyond any drought: root causes of chronic vulnerability in the Sahel', in *The Sahel Working Group*. Available at: http://www.iied.org/mediaroom /releases/070711sahel.html.

UNDP (2008), 'Indigenous knowledge in disaster management in Africa', in *United Nations Development Programme.* Available at: http://www.unep.org/IK/PDF/IndigenousBooklet.pdf.

UNEP (2010), 'Adapt Cost: Economics of climate change adaptation in Africa's water sector'. Available at: www.unep.org/climatechange/.../12%20AdaptCost%20water%report20FINAL.docX.

Urama, K.V. and Ozor, N. (2010), 'Impacts of climate change on water resources in Africa: the role of adaptation', in *Africa Technology Policy Studies Network.* Available at: http://www. ourplanet.com/climate-adap tation/Urama_Ozorv.pdf.

WWF (2006), 'Climate change impacts on east Africa: a review of the scientific literature', in World Wide Fund for Nature Climate Change Discussion Paper.

Chapter 8

Treatment of the Wastewater Containing Phenol and Strontium Using Isolated Cultures from Mine Water

Bilainu O. Oboirien

1. Introduction

Wastewater containing organic radioactive compounds is produced by the nuclear, medical, industrial, agricultural, and food processing industries either as part of the product or as a by product of the manufacturing process. The uncontrolled release of radioactive wastes from the above mentioned activities still poses many problems to human life and the natural environment due to its toxicity and the long half-lives of the radioisotopes in the waste (Zakrzewska-Trznadel, 2003). These wastes require treatment to meet discharge regulations to the inland waterways and to minimise the volume of radioactive material to be stored.

The presence of organic pollutants in a radioactive waste can interfere with the removal of the radionuclide (Yong *et al.* 2004; Chitra *et al.* 2004). Yong *et al.* (2004) reported that the presence of surfactants in a radioactive wastewater containing ^{241}Am (Amercium-241) had a great influence on the removal of ^{241}Am in a combined flocculation-microfiltration process. Without pretreatment of the surfactant, the radioactivity of ^{241}Am in the effluent was 316.6 Bq/l and a decontamination factor (DF) of 3.98. However, after the pretreatment of surfactants with potassium permanganate, the process produced an effluent with 1.0 Bq/l and a DF of 1651.4. Hence there is a need to treat the organic pollutant before the treatment of the radionuclides. The irradiated organic pollutants, even if not severely radioactive, are mostly recalcitrant in nature. For a successful bioremediation of an organic radioactive waste, biodegradation of the organic component has been identified as an initial step (Lange *et al.* 1998).

Microorganisms already living in contaminated environments are often well adapted to survival in the presence of existing contaminants and the temperature, pH, and oxidation potential of the site. Hence, microorganisms were isolated from uranium/gold mining water in South Africa. This study reports the degrading of an organic pollutant in a radioactive wastewater using isolated cultures from a gold mine in South Africa. Phenol and strontium, a major radionuclide found in low-level liquid radioactive waste was used to stimulate the organic radioactive wastewater. Radionuclides are potentially toxic to microorganisms on account of their chemical and radiological activity (Reed *et al.* 1999; Ruggiero *et al.* 2005). Future studies will involve the study of other organic compounds such as p-hydroxythmethylphenol, a binder used in the nuclear industry and phosphonated polystyrene ion exchange resin Purolite S-950 used in the production of medical radionuclide, ^{82} Sr(Strontium -82). In this study, only the chemical toxicity on the microorganisms is present since the simulated organic radioactive lacks radioactivity but contains similar chemical composition of the radioactive waste.

2. Materials and Methods

Reagents

Sr(NO3)2 arsenzo III reagent having an oxidation state of +2 (Sr^{2+}). Phenol and Folin-Ciocalteu phenol reagent were all purchased from

Sigma. All other chemicals were of analytical grade either from Merck or Fluka.

Enrichment of cultures

All microbial enrichment and isolation procedures were performed in nutrient broth containing (per litre): peptone 5g, NaCl 8 g, meat extract 1g, yeast extract containing 50 mg/L phenol. The mine water was collected from a gold mine in Gauteng, South Africa. 10ml of mine water was added into the flask containing 90 ml of the nutrient medium and 50 mg/L of phenol. The mixture was incubated in a lateral incubator shaker (Labcon SPL-M15) at an agitation rate of 120 rpm at 28°C. Optimum growth temperature will be determined in further studies. The biodegradation of phenol in the flask was monitored periodically with a UV/VIS spectrophotometer (WPA, Light Wave II, Labotech, South Africa). Nutrient broth was used in the enrichment studies because there was microbial no growth in the basic mineral medium.

Isolation of bacteria

About 10 ml of aliquot from the enrichment flask was spread on agar plated after serial dilutions for obtaining individual colonies of different bacteria. The plates were incubated at 28°C for 24 hours and colonies were carefully observed for their uniformity. The loopfuls of single colonies from each plate were streaked onto other fresh agar plates to check for purity.

Biodegradation tests

The phenol degradation capability of the isolated cultures under radionuclide exposure conditions was investigated in batch systems comprised of 500 ml Erlenmeyer flasks containing 100 ml of culture in a basal mineral medium. Simple media was used for the biodegradation test as opposed to the nutrient broth that was used for the enrichment studies because in our earlier study, there was accumulation of a brown colour compound during the biodegradation of phenol. This colour compounds might be an intermediate of phenol degradation. The partial degradation of phenol in the pure cultures used may be due to the existence of other more easily degradable carbon sources coming from the nutrient broth. The preliminary experimental design is presented in Table 1. Samples of 3 ml were taken aseptically at regular intervals. All tests were carried out in triplicate.

Table 1: Experimental design

Test	Properties
1	100 mg/L Phenol: 100 mg/L Strontium
2	200 mg/L Phenol: 200 mg/L Strontium
3	300 mg/L Phenol: 300 mg/L Strontium
4	500 mg/L Phenol: 500 mg/L Strontium
Control	200 mg/L Phenol: 200 mg/L Strontium without cells

Analytical methods

Cell growth was monitored by measuring the optical density (OD) of the culture in a UV/VIS spectrophotometer (WPA, Light Wave II, Labotech, South Africa) at 600 nm. The cell density was confirmed by dry weight analysis. Phenol concentration was determined using the Folin-Ciocalteu reagent and was confirmed by HPLC.

Qualitative analysis of phenol was determined colorimetrically using the Folin-Ciocalteu Method (Box, 1983). The sensitivity and the detection limit of this method are 8 mg/L and 5mg/L 1 ml of sample solution or standard solution was added to 10 ml of distilled water and 1.0 ml of Folin-Ciocalteu reagent. The mixture was allowed to stand for 5 minutes and then 2.0 ml of sodium carbonate was added to the mixture. After 1 hour in a dark place the absorbance nm was measured at 750 nm in a UV/VIS spectrophotometer (WPA, Light Wave II, Labotech, South Africa).

Phenol and metabolites was made using were analyzed in an HPLC (Hewlett Packard Agilent 1100 series) with DAD detection (diode array detector, 280, 325, 340 nm). A Luna 3u C-18 (Phenomenex®) reverse phase column (250 mm by 4.6 mm) was used. A gradient elution was performed with water (pH 2.6 adjusted with H3PO4) and acetonitrile (ACN) as follows: 0 min, 7% ACN; 0 – 20 min, 20% ACN; 20 – 28 min, 23% ACN; 28 – 40 min, 27%, ACN; 40 – 45 min, 29%, ACN; 45 – 47 min, 33%, ACN. The flow rate was 1 ml/min, and the injection volume was 20 µl. This equipment is located in the Department of Plant Science at the University of Pretoria, South Africa.

3. Results and Discussion

Isolation of phenol degrading cultures

Microorganisms are known to have evolved several biochemical pathways for degrading or transforming a variety of toxic compounds either for survival in hostile environments or for energy conservation. This is especially the case when the microorganisms are exposed to the same compound or class of compounds for prolonged periods. Hence, an effort was made to isolate and study microbial cultures from radiation exposed, contaminated soil or water environments. In this study, microorganisms were isolated from uranium/ gold mines effluent in Guateng, South Africa. The isolated cultures were able to degrade phenol in the presence of strontium in the simulated organic radioactive waste.

Phenol Degradation

The extent of phenol degradation by the isolated mine cultures at different initial phenol concentration is shown in Figure 1. The result shows that there was phenol biodegradation in the entire range of initial phenol concentration that was investigated in this study (100-500 mg/L). The degradation rate varied largely for the different initial concentrations. In all the batches, the degradation rate increased with incubation time. The highest maximum rate per batch appeared between 36 and 50 hours in the 500 mg/L. Hence there would be a need to increase the initial concentration above 500 mg/L.

The effect of initial phenol concentration on the growth of the isolated cultures is presented in Figure 2. Biomass concentration was monitored by measuring its absorbance at 600 nm and by dry weight analysis. From the curve in Figure 2, it was observed that the lag time of the cultures was prolonged and there was hardly any growth. This was confirmed from the results from the dry weight analysis. There was negligible increase in the total biomass weight after 48 hours of incubation. Another observation was that the time the maximum absorbance of the cultures was obtained for the different concentrations corresponds to the incubation time when complete degradation was also obtained for the different concentration of phenol.

Figure 1: Phenol degradation in batch culture experiment

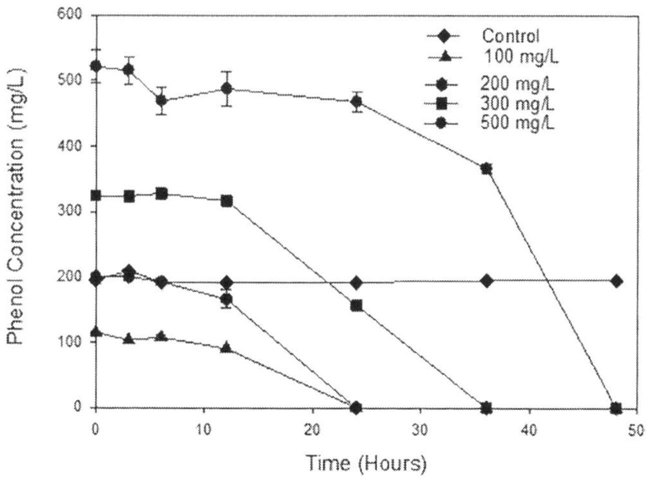

Figure 2: Optical density at 600 nm (OD_{600}) of the cultures as a function of time at different initial phenol concentration

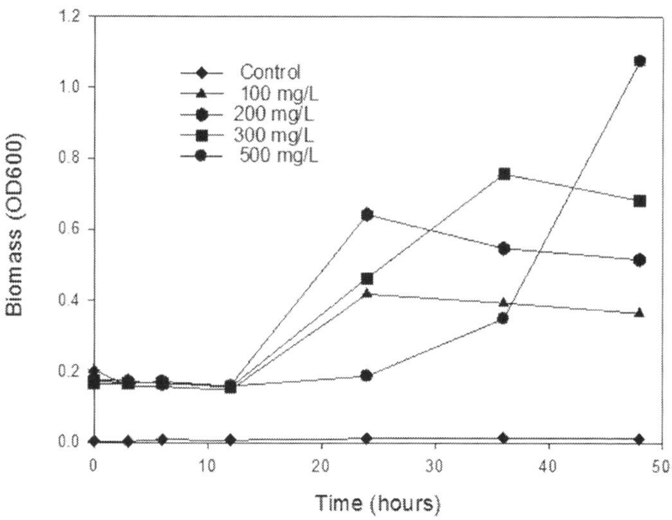

Metabolite Analysis

Metabolic intermediates may inhibit the biodegradation of organic aromatic compounds such as phenol. Extracts of the biodegraded sample were analysed using HPLC operations. The phenolic metabolites were identified on the basis of the chromatographic retention time of authentic compounds. The results for the 200 mg/L are shown in Figures 3 and 4. The retention times of the peaks indicate the presence of any compound (phenol and its metabolites), while the areas of the peaks give the amount of the various metabolites. The absence of phenolic peak at 32 mins in Figure 4 shows the disappearance of phenol and therefore confirms the results obtained using the using the Folin-Ciocalteu reagent. Similar data was also obtained for the different concentrations tested. Also the presence of a peak at 16 mins indicates the presence of an intermediate. This peak was also obtained in 100 mg/L, 300 mg/L and 500 mg/L. However it was absent in the controltest. These results suggest that the peak is a byproduct from the phenol biodegradation process.

The biodegradation of phenol resulted in the drop in pH. This is presented in Table 2. The drop in pH might be due to the accumulation of organic acids, which are possible intermediates from the biodegradation of phenol.

Table 2: Change in pH during biodegradation

Properties	Initial pH at 0 hours	Final pH at 48 hours
100 mg/L	6.68	5.83
200 mg/L	6.68	5.83
300 mg/L	6.68	5.68
500 mg/L	6.68	5.51
Control	6.68	6.68

Figure 3: HPLC results of 200 mg/L phenol at time 0 hours

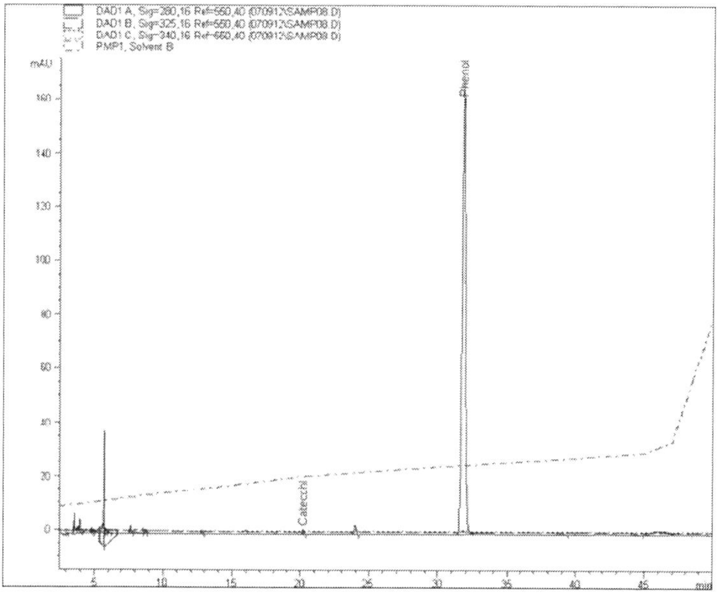

Figure 4: HPLC results of 200 mg/L at time 48 hours

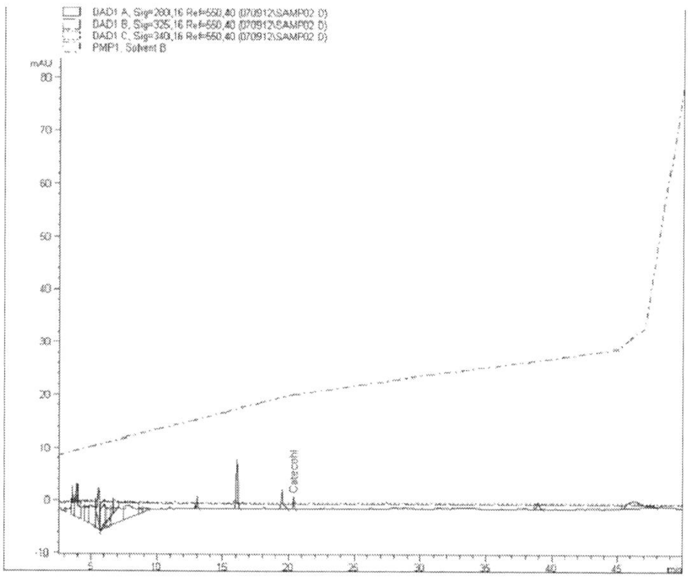

4. Conclusion

Phenol and strontium, a major radionuclide found in low-level liquid radioactive waste was used to simulate the organic radioactive wastewater. The cultures were grown on phenol ranging from 100-500 mg/L as the sole carbon source. The isolated cultures were able to degrade phenol of a maximum concentration of 500 mg/L in 48 hours. The highest maximum rate per batch appeared between 36 and 50 hours in the 500 mg/L, hence there would be a need to increase the initial concentration above 500 mg/L. The described culture and represents a significant contribution towards the decontamination efforts in environments contaminated with radioactive waste.

References

Box, J. D. (1983), 'Investigation of the Folin-Ciocalteau phenol reagent for the determination of polyphenolic substances in natural waters', in *Water Research*, 17: 511-525

Chitra, S., Paramasivan, K., Sinha, P.K. and Lal, K.B. (2004), 'Ultrasonic treatment of liquid waste containing EDTA', in *Journal of Cleaner Production,* 12: 429-435.

Lange, C., Wackett, L., Minton, K. and Daly, M.J. (1998), 'Engineering a recombinant *Dienonocuss radiodurans* for organopollutant degradation in radioactive mixed waste environments', in *Nature Biotechnology,* 16: 929-933.

Reed, D.T., Vojta, Y., Quinn, J.W. and Richmann, M.K. (1999), 'Radiotoxicity of plutonium NTA-degrading *Chelatobacter heintzii* cell suspensions', in *Biodegradation*, 10: 251- 260.

Ruggiero, C.E., Boukhalfa, H., Forsythe, J.H., Lack, J.G., Hersman, L.E. and Neu, M.P. (2005), 'Actinide and metal toxicity to prospective bioremediation bacteria', in *Environmental Microbiology,* 7: 88-97.

Yong, G., Jun, Z., Guanghui, Z., Dong, Z., Weiwen, Y., Xuejun, L., Bangzhong, M., Junhui, Z. and Ping, G. (2004), 'Treatment of the wastewater containing low-level ^{241}Am using flocculation-microfiltration process', in *Separation and Purification Technology*, 40: 183-189.

Zakrzewska-Trznadel, G. (2003), 'Radioactive solutions treatment by hybrid complexation- UF/NF process', in *Journal of Membrane Science*, 225: 25-39.

Chapter 9

Technical Challenges for Water Borehole Design, Construction and Maintenance in the Eastern Niger Delta of Nigeria

Nwankwoala, H.O. & Udom, G.J.

1. Introduction

The abstraction of groundwater in the Eastern Niger Delta is constantly faced with many challenges ranging from terrain difficulties, high iron contents, saline water intrusion, poor quality of groundwater in the riverine areas, uncertainty in the geology/ hydrogeology and quality of experienced manpower, lack of funds to execute complex drilling and abuse of practice (Etu- Efeotor & Odigi (1983); Amadi & Amadi (1990); Amajor (1986); Amadi, *et al.*, (1989); Etu-Efeotor, (1981); Udom, *et al.*, (1999); Nwaogazie, (2006); Nwankwoala, *et al.*, (2007); Nwankwoala & Udom (2008); Nwankwoala & Udom (2011a); Nwankwoala & Udom, 2011b).

In the Eastern Niger Delta, and indeed much of the country,

groundwater exploration precedes any local or regional groundwater resource management as it provides pre-drilling information useful in borehole designs (Amajor, 1989). This important preliminary phase to borehole construction is rarely carried out and where it is done only scanty information is available.

The increasing stress on the groundwater due to competing needs of humans and other users of water as well as the high and increasing pollution potentials in the study area underscore the great need to constantly and adequately train people for operation, maintenance and management of water supply systems. This will assure not only the continued existence of the groundwater at source but also the functionality and acceptability of water supply systems in the future. This paper maintains that it is one thing to construct a water supply facility and another to sustain it. This paper therefore argues that it is absolutely important that groundwater resource needs to be handled in a sustainable manner so as to align the study area with the UN-driven Millennium Development Goals (MDGs).

Borehole has remained one major source for water supply in parts of the Niger Delta. Year in, year out, governments at all levels as well as private organizations and individuals construct boreholes in the area. But despite the reported success of these projects and numerous programmes, meeting safe water needs has remained poor. So many agitating questions have remained unanswered. Is it that these boreholes are not enough or they are not providing services for a long time? What is the life span of a borehole? These and related questions are addressed in this paper, especially as groundwater is the sure source of potable water in the study area.

2. Brief geology/hydrogeology of the study area

The Eastern Niger Delta covers most areas of Rivers and Bayelsa States (Figure 1). Geologically, the study area is characterized by the Niger Delta sedimentary rocks. Lithostratigraphically, these rocks are divided into the oldest Akata Formation (Paleocene), the Agbada Formation (Eocene) and the Youngest Benin Formation (Miocene to Recent). Generally, the present knowledge of the geology of the Niger Delta was derived from the works of the following researchers

(Reyment, 1965; Short & Stauble, 1967; Murat, 1970; Merki, 1970) as well as the exploration activities of the oil and gas companies in Nigeria. The formation of the so called proto-Niger Delta occurred during the second depositional cycle (Campanian-Maastrichtian) of the southern Nigerian basin. However, the modern Niger Delta was formed during the third and last depositional cycle of the southern Nigerian basin which started in the Paleocene.

The geologic sequence of the Niger Delta consists of three main tertiary subsurface lithostratigraphic units (Short & Stauble, 1967) which are overlain by various types of Quaternary deposits (Table 1).

Table 1: Quaternary deposits of the Niger Delta (after Etu-Efeotor & Akpokodje, 1990)

Geologic Unit	Lithology	Age
Alluvium	Gravel, Sand, clay, silt	Quaternary
Freshwater Backswamp, meander belt	Sand, clay, some silt, gravel	
Saltwater Mangrove Swamp and backswamp	Medium-fine sands, clay and some silt	
Active/abandoned beach ridges	Sand, clay, and some silt	
Sombreiro-warri deltaic plain	Sand, clay, and some silt	

Figure 1: Location Map of the Study Area (Modified after Amajor, 1986)

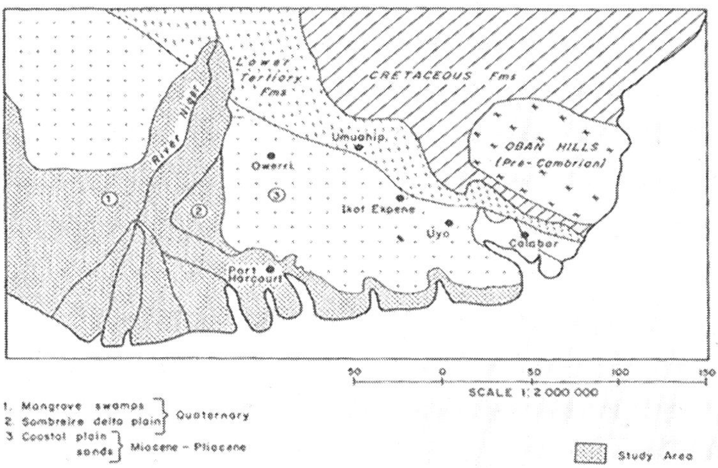

Hydrogeologically, the major aquiferous formation in the study area is the Benin Formation. It is about 2100m thick at the basin centre and consists of coarse-medium grained sandstones, thick shales and gravels. The upper section of the Benin Formation is the quaternary deposits which is about 40 – 150m thick and comprises of sand and silt/clay with the later becoming increasingly more prominent seawards (Etu-Efeotor & Akpokodje, 1990). The formation consists of predominantly freshwater continental friable sands and gravel that have excellent aquifer properties with occasional intercalations of claystone/shales (Olobaniyi & Owoyemi, 2006). According to Etu-Efeotor (1981), Etu-Efeotor & Akpokodje (1990), Offodile (2002), Udom *et al* (2002), the Benin Formation is highly permeable, prolific, productive and is the most extensivelytapped aquifer in the Niger Delta. All the boreholes in the study area are drilled into it. The Benin Formation consists of fluvial and lacustrine deposits whose thicknesses are variable but generally exceed 1970 meters (Asseez, 1989). The lithologies of the Benin Formation include sands, silts, gravel and clayey intercalations. The sands are fine to coarse-grained, gravelly, poorly sorted and sub-angular to well rounded.

According to Onyeagocha (1980), the rocks of the Benin Formation are made up of about 95 – 99% quartz grains, Na+K – Mica 1 -2.5%, feldspar 0.5 1.0% and dark minerals 2.3%. These minerals are loosely bound by calcite and silica cement. The clayey intercalations have given rise to multi-aquifer systems in the area. The main source of recharge is through direct precipitation where annual rainfall is as high as 2000 – 2400mm. The water infiltrates through the highly permeable sands of the Benin Formation to recharge the aquifers. Groundwater in the study area occurs principally under water table conditions. Multi-aquifer systems occur in the study area and the upper aquifers are generally unconfined (Etu-Efeotor, 1981; Offodile, 2002; Edet, 1993; and Udom, 2004).

The study area consists of a broad riverine area through which the River Niger enters the Atlantic, divided into numerous rivulets which fan out into the sea. It also includes a number of tidal creeks separating small islands of less than 10m above sea level (Offodile, 1992).

Generally, the most important aquifers in the Niger Delta are the Deltaic and Benin Formations. Most of the boreholes in the northern parts of the Niger Delta tap unconfined aquifers. In most of the boreholes, the geological sequence consists of continuous sandy formations from top to bottom (Adelana *et al.*, 2008). However, some of the aquifers occur under confined conditions, resulting in artesian flows. The marked distinction between Deltaic and Benin Formation are briefly highlighted below.

Unconfined Aquifers of the Deltaic Formation

The water table is very close to the ground surface, ranging from 0-9m below ground level. The aquifers in this area obtain steady recharge through direct precipitation and major rivers. Rainfall in the Delta is heavy, varying from about 2400mm a year inland to 4800mm near the coast. Some proportion of the rainfall is lost by runoff and evapotranspiration. NEDECO (1961) recorded 720 – 960 mm/a of evapotranspiration along the coast, which is mainly thick mangrove swamps, to 1200mm/a in the northern parts of the delta which is less thickly vegetated. Hence, very limited water table fluctuation is expected in these areas where there is heavy rainfall nearly all the year round. According to Offodile (1992), the Deltaic Plains (Late Pleistocene to Holocene in age) have specific capacities in the range 160 320 m^3/d/m.

Confined Aquifers of the Benin Formation

The sediments of the Benin Formation are more permeable than those of the Deltaic Plains. The depth to water table ranges between 3 and 15m below ground surface. A few values for seasonal fluctuations obtained from the area, indicate seasonal differences between 2.1 and 3.6m. The Benin Formation is sandy and highly permeable (Nwankwoala & Udom, 2011a), with specific capacity 150 and 1400 m^3/d/m (Offodile, 1992). Confined aquifers occur within both the Deltaic Formation and Benin Formation. These formations are characterized by moderately high yielding artesian flows. In some areas, the aquifers are confined by a shale or clay bed up to 36 m thick. The total depth of the aquifers below this shale bed is not yet determined.

However, borehole data indicate a depth of approximately 100 m. Hydrogeological information indicates a hydrological connection between the confined aquifers along the coastline and the unconfined aquifers of the Benin Formation to the north, inland (Ngerebara & Nwankwoala, 2008). The aquifers increase in thickness towards the mainland, while the confining clays thin out. The specific capacity for this formation varies from 90 – 320 m^3/d/m. In the area underlain by the Benin Formation, the confined aquifers occur in the southern part of the Niger Delta. The aquifer was confined by several shale and clay beds. The specific capacity for this formation varies between 140 and 180 m3/d/m, and artesian flows have been measured up to 6 l/s (Adelana *et al.,* 2008).

3. Evolution of groundwater in the study area

The evolution of the groundwater in the study area can be explained by the order of encounter as stated by Freeze & Cherry (1979). The theory states that the order in which groundwaters encounter strata of different mineraological compositions can exert an important control on the final water chemistry. As groundwater flows through strata of different mineralogical composition, the water composition undergoes adjustments caused by imposition of new mineralogically controlled thermodynamic constraints.

Basically, the Niger Delta water resources are drawn from the Eastern littoral, hydrological and the Niger South hydrological zones. Infiltration and percolation processes from these broad recharge network flow southwards into the underlying aquifers of the Benin Formation beneath the Continental Shelf (Ngerebara & Nwankwoala, 2008). Both the structural and stratigraphic setting of the Niger Delta favours hydraulic gradient flow towards the coast and hence into the Continental Shelf. This forms the basis of most freshwater aquifers located within the Continental Shelf. The general rainfall pattern in the Niger Delta ensures a permanent supply of water to the region.

4. Factors responsible for borehole lifespan

Many factors are responsible for the life span of a borehole in the study area. In order to effectively construct a good borehole expected to render years of satisfactory performance, so many considerations are to be put in place at the planning stage. Though, some of the factors are directly under the control of owner/client, while at the same time, other pertinent factors are under the control of the driller/contractor. Construction, completion and development; operations and maintenance; and other factors largely control the life span of a borehole.

Construction, completion and development

Hydraulic percussion, cable tool, mechanical and hydraulic rotary (normal and reverse circulation), and combined percussion-rotary are some of the effective drilling methods used in groundwater exploration. In each of the methods highlighted above, the choice of a particular method depends on the purpose for which the borehole is to serve, the characteristics of the rocks as well as the quality of water required, depth to aquifer, in addition to ancillary factors such as cost factors and technical factors (honesty of the driller).

Because the sands of the Benin Formation are unconsolidated, the conventional rotary method which is faster and highly economical is widely used in majority of the Eastern Niger Delta. Mobile truck mounted hydraulic and mechanical (tripod) rigs are used in dry upland (upper delta) and swampy (lower delta) areas, respectively, because of the inherent transportation problems dictated by the terrain (Amajor, 1989). Though, the tripod rig method is a good drilling practice, the technique requiresa good choice of drill bit, stem and fluid which is dictated by the geologic conditions to be encountered in the area. Inadequate knowledge can lead to hole collapse, stuck drilling pipes, well development problems, poor sample recovery and more importantly, unusual longer drilling time (common in the study area, especially with the tripod method of drilling).

It is important to know the purpose to which a borehole is to serve, the expected yield of the borehole based on whether it is going to provide sustainable water all the time for a household, a block of few flats, a residential estate, a community/town, a factory or municipal water works? It is important to know that the expected yield and location leads to the choice of pump type, well diameter, screen length as well as depth range, having in mind the static water level (SWL) and hydrogeology of the area.

The choice of the pump type determines the final casing diameter while the final casing diameter determines the open hole diameter, having in mind an annulus of 2 – 3 inches to allow for free casing installation and appropriate thickness of gravel packing and/or grouting.

Well completion involves screening the intake section of the aquifer, casing the remaining portion of the well up to a few feet above ground level and well development. If these are properly designed, they make for not only excellent yield but also long life of the well. The choice of completion materials i.e casing, screen and gravel) used in the completion of a borehole plays an important role in the life span of the well. Most people are not aware that casings, for instance, are of different thickness or schedules while screen are also of different collapse pressures as well as slot sizes. Normally, appropriate well casing and screen must resist substantial compressive, tensile and collapsing forces and should last for 20 – 40 years when in contact with soil on the outside and water/humid atmosphere on the inside.

Borehole depth as well as the quality of water can play a significant role in the choice of completion materials. Aggressive corrosion, heavy incrustation or both often suggest use of special alloys, non-metallic pipes or special coating of low carbon steel pipes for use as casings (Konyebagu, 2009; Udom & Acra, 2006). Coatings may not be the choice. This is because it is practically impossible to install a casing without breaking the coating on the outside of the casing by abrasion or to install a pump without breaking the coating on the inside of the casing. Where the coating is broken often becomes a point of aggressive concentrated corrosion attack, hence, the choice of completion materials based on predetermined mindset are as follows:

(a) Ceramic Clay and Concrete Pipes

These materials are not only resistant to corrosion but could also be subject to some attack and are unsatisfactory if a well is acidized. More importantly, they are very heavy in weight and difficult to install and keep in alignment as their joints are difficult to make tightly sealed up. Due to their weight and strength characteristics, deep installation or setting may result in compressive failure of the pipe at the bottom, hence, only commonly used in hand dug shallow wells.

(b) Asbestos cement pipes

These are lighter somehow more resistant than concrete with respect to corrosion. They are also available in longer lengths and special joint seals are available. However, these pipes present many of the problems associated with concrete pipe and also been reported to impact negatively on the quality as well as public health.

(c) Plastic Pipes

Plastic pipes such as Poly vinyl chloride (PVC), Polyethylene, Acrylonitrile – Butadiene – Styrene (ABS) or Rubber modified plastics offer many advantages such as light weight, ease of fabrication, corrosion and acid resistance and low price. They are easily available in appropriate length, wall thickness and diameter. It is also difficult to join it with steel pipes. They have been successfully used for wells up to 100 – 120m.

(d) Fibre Glass Reinforced Plastic Pipes

These have been used extensively in water supply even up to about 80m. However, the conditions are exceptional and its collapse under normal development procedures has been reported to be a problem. The pipes offer all the advantages of plastic pipe plus greater collapse strength except for the higher cost.

(e) Stainless Steel and Various Copper Alloys

These are satisfactory from nearly all standpoints as well as casing. However, they are expensive and justifiable only in permanent wells in very corrosive environments.

The casing (pipes of various sizes and composition used to protect the unscreened portion of the well from collapse which serves as a housing for the pump and a conduit for water flow upwards to the surface). Casing sizes is dictated by the bowl size of the pump and expected water yield and water quality. Water contamination can occur through corrosion of any part of the casing (WHO, 2003). The collapse resistance of pipe increases with the wall thickness, the elasticity and the yield strength of the material and decreases with an increase in pipe diameter. From all standpoints, except corrosion resistance, low carbon steel pipe is the most satisfactory material for use as well casing. In their installation, they can be threaded, welded, brazed or even the three (3) together to ensure tightness, safety and durability. Studies have also shown that doubling the wall thickness of a steel pipe extends the life of the pipe about four times.

In most parts of the eastern Niger Delta, API steel, inferior galvanized steel and plastic pipes have been used in places. However, the choice of casing diameter is usually not based on the expected yield. The use of very cheap and inferior casing materials has contaminated lots of boreholes (Amajor, 1989). This, in turn has given rise to many pumps being lost in the hole.

Gravel packing (introduction of artificially graded siliceous gravels around the screen to make the area more permeable thereby increasing the effective diameter of the well) is conducted for thick artesian, unconsolidated, uniform fine sand and laminated aquifers. The grading of the gravel is selected on the basis of the results of grain size distribution study on the aquifer samples. The size of the screen slot is then controlled by the size of the gravel (Johnson, 1975). In the study area, gravel packing is commonly practiced. However, the sizes of the gravel as well as screen slot widths are not based on the results of mechanical analysis of aquifer and gravel samples. Such a practice has caused considerable borehole development problems for many water drilling contractors in the study area (Amajor, 1989).

Operations and Maintenance

After a satisfactory borehole completion exercise, the operation and maintenance become very important. With proper operation and regular maintenance, a borehole is expected to last up to 50 or more years. Regular and proper maintenance of a borehole is important as it helps to prevent or pre-empt problems such as: dropping of pump, clogging of screen, accumulation of silt, clearing of rust, corrosion and incrustation. It is very desirable and necessary that the client/

well owner maintain a proper log book where the well performances as well as the general observations are recorded. Such records should normally be made available for inspection and possible interpretation to the professional for appropriate action (Konyebagu, 2009).

It is important to note that no matter how small a problem, immediate action should be taken to salvage the situation otherwise such solvable problem could end up as a major problem. For example, due to lack of servicing, a pump can drop into a well. Another pump can be installed to allow for continued functioning with good yield. Routine flushing/airlifting can be carried out on boreholes. This is very important because failure to service water systems over long period of time may result in any or combination of the following, according to Nwaogazie (2006):

i) Clogging of borehole screen;

ii) Impaired flow (reduction in borehole yield);

iii) Silting of the borehole;

iv) Deposit of sediments on the pump, borehole casings and risers;

v) Corrosion of any metal surface (pump, household appliances);

vi) Sediment trapping in pump resulting in impaired pumping and pump failure;

vii) Impaired pumping resulting from leaking risers (increase in tank-filling time);

viii) Deposit of sediments I storage tanks;

ix) Presence of micro-organisms (including algae) in storage tanks;

x) Presence of odour and taste in water caused by the activity of micro-organisms;

xi) Occurrence of water-borne diseases; and

xii) Wearing of borehole components ultimately leading to facility breakdown.

Other factors

Other factors such as costs and appropriate pricing and honesty of the driller play a major role. There have been many cases where a client briefs the contractor on how much he wants to spend to drill a borehole. The contractor then chose the type of materials suitable for the offered price but may not be suitable for durability/sustainability of the borehole. Most often, when a tender becomes very competitive based on pricing, especially where there are so many loopholes on the bill of quantities in terms of defining the type of materials required, the desire to get the job becomes the contractor's main purpose and this pushes quality and durability to second position, giving rise to a lot of things that will eventually compromise the life span of the borehole. The driller and the client need to keep accurate log and observations of the well performance. Though not a technical factor, it has become very important in considering the life span of a borehole.

It is interesting to note that many contractors are known to have problems during borehole construction or completion. Sometimes the problems can be satisfactorily solved but either they lack the knowledge or the resources to do it right. For instance, after the wrong choice of screen slot e.g. say slot 020 in a fine sand aquifer, the borehole should be assisted with very thorough backwashing and good grade of gravel packing. Unfortunately, after casing installation, as per well design, the mud pump could not carry out the necessary backwashing for which reason the exercise of gravel packing was pushed forward to allow for repair of the pump. By the time the pump is repaired, the borehole had collapsed and proper gravel packing could not be achieved. A situation of this nature would require patience and prolonged development as alternate jetting and airlifting would have to be done for a long time to enable the hole undergo natural gravel packing. But due to lack of knowledge, resources and equipment, the contractor hires a compressor and airlift for 2 -4 hours and returns the compressor thereafter. The final well discharge has significant amount of fine sand and mud, yet the well was declared as successful to the client. Naturally, such a well would not last for long before parking up and would require this information for another contractor to quote appropriately and restore the well.

In the study area, compressed air is commonly used for borehole development. In a few cases jetting with water at high velocity has been successful. Both methods are acceptable but the latter is more effective, and advantageous. Because of the poor screen design, development has been unsuccessful in many boreholes in the study area. It is important to note that a successful development program depends more on a better screen design that is geologically controlled. There are so many cases of materials or tools dropping into the well and abandoned without reporting to client or casing installation not getting to designed depth with screens not properly set in the aquifer, yet well is declared as successful and commissioned. Most often, contractors are not honest enough to report such mishap and would not even on their own try to solve the problem satisfactorily before hurriedly handing the job over to the client.

Another dimension on the honest factor is the contractor's willingness not to engage in sharp, unethical or unprofessional practices. Sometimes the client has been charged and made to pay for the appropriate materials but the contractor being dishonest plays on his ignorance and deliberately completes the well with substandard and cheap materials. There are also cases where the contractor would honestly buy what he believes to be the best at the price of the superior materials, unknown to him that the materials (screen/pumps/electrical component/cable, etc) are indeed not the one he intended but only well packaged with false labels by the dealer and sold to him as the genuine and standard materials. This paper advocates that such sharp practices by both contractors and dealer must stop for successful delivery of boreholes.

5. Conclusion

Borehole construction and maintenance in parts of the eastern Niger Delta has become very unfavourable to both client and contractors alike. More importantly, contractors must ensure that materials bought for any project is checked and tested before use. It is also very necessary that client understands that a relatively cheap option has its own cost.

The high level of quackery in the practice, with the result that despite huge sums of fund invested, non conformity with standards and specifications results in poorly completed wells. Poorly constructed boreholes as well as those in areas of high groundwater pollution potentials should be serviced at least twice a year. More so the fluctuating nature of borehole drilling materials goes with the trend of the economy and borehole materials for efficient service delivery of water supply should be supported by both government and private sector.

References

Adelana, S.M.A., Olasehinde, P.I., Bale, R.B., Vrbka, P., Edet, A.E. and Goni, I.B. (2008), 'An overview of the Geology and Hydrogeology of Nigeria', In: Adelana, S.M.A. and MacDonald, A.M. (eds.), *Applied Groundwater Studies in Africa, Selected Papers on Hydrogeology*. CRC Press/Balkema, The Netherlands.

Amadi P.A., Ofoegbu, C.O. and Morrison, T. (1989), 'Hydrogeochemical assessment of groundwater quality in parts of the Niger Delta, Nigeria', in *Environmental Geology Water Science*, 14(3): 195- 202.

Amadi, U.M.P. and Amadi, P.A. (1990), 'Saltwater migration in the coastal aquifers of southern Nigeria', in *Journal of Mining and Geology,* 26(1):35-44

Amajor, L.C. (1986), 'Alluvial fan facies in the Miocene-Pliocene coastal plain sands, Niger Delta, Nigeria', in *Sedimentary Geology*, 49:1-20

Amajor, L.C. (1989), 'Geological appraisal of groundwater exploitation in the Eastern Niger Delta', In: Ofoegbu, C.O. (ed.), *Groundwater and Mineral Resources of Nigeria*, Braunschweig/ Weisbaden, Friedr Vieweg and Sohn.

Asseez, L.O. (1989), 'Review of the stratigraphy, sedimentation and structure of the Niger Delta' In: Kogbe, C.A. (ed.), *Geology of Nigeria*, Rockview Nigeria Limited.

Edet, A.E. (1993), 'Groundwater quality assessment in parts of Eastern Niger Delta, Nigeria', in *Environmental Geology*, 22:41-46

Etu-Efeotor, J.O. (1981), 'Preliminary hydrogeochemical investigation of subsurface waters in parts of the Niger Delta', in *Journal of Mining and Geology*. 18(1):103-105.

Etu-Efeotor, J.O. and Akpokodje, E.G. (1990), 'Aquifer systems of the Niger Delta', in *Journal of Mining Geology,* 26(2):279 – 284.

Etu-Efeotor, J.O. and Odigi, M.I. (1983), 'Water supply problems in the Eastern Niger Delta', in *Journal of Mining and Geology,* 26(2):279-279.

Freeze, R.A. and Cherry, J.A. (1979), '*Groundwater',* Englewood Cliffs, NJ: Prentice Hall.

Johnson, E.E (1975), '*Groundwater and Wells'*, Johnson Division UOP Inc., Minnesota.

Konyebagu, R. (2009), 'What is the life span of a borehole?', in *Water Front Bulletin of the Nigeria Water and Sanitation Association*, 10: 33 – 35.

Merki, J.P. (1970), 'Structural geology of the Cenozoic Niger Delta', In: Dessauvagie, T.T J and Whiteman, A.J (eds.), *African Geology*, University of Ibadan Press, Ibadan, Nigeria African Geology, University of Ibadan Press.

Murat, R.C. (1970), '*Stratigraphy and paleogeography of the cretaceous and lower tertiary in southern Nigeria'*, In: Dessauvagie, T.T J and Whiteman, A.J (eds.), *African Geology*, University of Ibadan Press, Ibadan, Nigeria.

NEDECO (Netherlands Engineering Company) (1961), '*River studies and recommendations on improvement on the Niger and Benue*', North Holland Publishing Company.

Ngerebara, O.D. and Nwankwoala, H.O. (2008), 'Groundwater resources potential in the offshore Niger Delta, Nigeria', in '*Journal of Environmental Hydrology'*, Paper 28.

Nwankwoala, H.O., Okeke, E.V. and Okereke, S.C. (2007), 'Groundwater quality in parts of Port Harcourt, Nigeria: an overview, trends and concerns', in *International Journal of Biotechnology and Allied Sciences*, 2(3): 282-289.

Nwankwoala , H.O. and Udom, G.J. (2008), 'Influence of land reclamation on the status of groundwater in Borokiri area of Port Harcourt, Niger Delta, Nigeria', in *International Journal of Natural and Applied Sciences,* 4(4):431-434.

Nwankwoala, H.O. and Udom, G.J. (2011a), 'A preliminary review of potential groundwater resources of the Niger Delta', in *Inter-*

national Journal of Applied Environmental Sciences, 6(1):57-70.

Nwankwoala, H.O. and Udom, G.J. (2011b), ' Hydrochemical facies and Ionic ratios of groundwater in Port Harcourt, southern Nigeria', in *Research Journal of Chemical Sciences,* 1(3): 87-101.

Nwaogazie, I.L. (2006), 'Water supply for all: who cares', *Inaugural Lecture Series*, No 52, University of Port Harcourt, July 27, 2006.

Offodile, M.E. (1992), *A approach to groundwater study and development in Nigeria*, Mecon, Jos, Nigeria.

Offodile, M.E. (2002), *Groundwater study and development in Nigeria*, Mecon Eng. Servies Ltd, Jos, Nigeria.

Olobaniyi, S.B. and Owoyemi, F.B. (2006), 'Characterization by factor analysis of the chemical facies of groundwater in the Deltaic plain sands aquifers of Warri, Western Niger Delta, Nigeria', in *African Journal of Science and Technology, Science and Engineering Series,* 7(1):73-81.

Onyeagocha, A.C. (1980), 'The petrology and depositional environment of the Benin formation', in *Nigerian Journal of Mining and Geology,* 17(2):147-151.

Reyment, R.A. (1965), '*Aspects of geology of Nigeria'*, University of Ibadan Press, Nigeria.

Short, K.C. and Stauble, A.J. (1967), 'Outline of the geology of the Niger Delta', in *Bulletin, AAPG*, 51:761-779.

Udom, G.J. (2004), 'Regional hydrogeology of Akwa Ibom State, Nigeria, using lithological, pump testing and resistivity data', *Unpublished Ph.D Thesis*, University of Calabar, Nigeria.

Udom, G.J., Etu-Efeotor, J.O. and Esu, E.O. (1999), 'Hydrogeochemical characteristics of groundwater in parts of Port Harcourt and Tai-Eleme Local Government Areas', in *Global Journal of Pure and Applied Sciences,* 5(5):545-552.

Udom, G.J., Ushie, F.A. and Esu, E.O (2002), 'A geochemical survey of groundwater in Khana and Gokana Local Government

Areas of Rivers State', in *Journal of Applied Science and Environmental Management,* 6(1): 53-59

Udom, G.J. and Acra, E.J. (2006), 'Hydrochemical characteristics of groundwater in Andoni Local Governemt Area, Rivers State', in *Journal of Research in Physical Sciences,* 2(1):35-41

WHO (2003), 'Water supply, sanitation and hygiene development, water sanitation and health'. Available at http://www.who.int/water_sanitation/health/hygiene/en/

Chapter 10

Reflections on Water and Wellbeing:

The Political Imperatives in Nigeria

Segun Oshewolo, Angathevar Baskaran &
Mammo Muchie

1. Introduction

The essentiality of water to human wellbeing has received ample theoretical and empirical attention (Novo, 2012; Mobie and Masango, 2009; Martins, 2001; United Nations Environment Programme, 2009). Water has been called the 'berth of life' as it performs basic ecological functions in every environment. It is the most important molecule for both biosphere and society (Novo, 2012: 65). Humans are heavily dependent on water for their sustenance. They can survive longer without food than without water and he requires water for drinking, cooking, washing, sanitation, farming, and factory use (Ayoade, 1975: 581). Water is therefore fundamental to the health of the biosphere, strong economic growth and human social wellbeing (Carter, 2007: 330). Apropos of the foregoing, individuals, national governments, and concerned international bodies have been striving to promote access to good water. However, in terms of performance, variations exist across the globe. While the performance of some countries has been consistently admirable, the same cannot be said concerning African countries. They have consistently been ranked as countries with the least sustainable access to improved water sources such as piped water into dwelling, yard or plot, public tap or standpipe, tubewell or borehole, protected spring, and hygienic collection of rain water (Africa Public Health, 2012).

The situation in Nigeria is harrowing. In 2006, national good water coverage failed to improve across Nigeria. Instead it fell from 49 per cent in 1990 to 48 per cent in 2004 (Oshewolo and Oniemola, 2011: 262; Integrated Regional Information Network, 2007). The World Health Organisation and UNICEF report for 2012 ranked Nigeria third behind China and India, as countries with the largest population without adequate water and sanitation. This is a critical challenge given the fact that women and children trek long distances to fetch water from streams and ponds which are most times contaminated (Daily Times NG, May 12, 2012). According to Nigeria's Honourable Minister of Water Resources, Mrs Sarah Ochekpe, the current water supply service coverage in the country is 58 per cent, which represents about 87 million people. This translates to lack of potable water for about 70 million people. The situation is more frightening in the rural areas. Only 42 per cent have access to potable water supply in the rural areas (Punch, February 24, 2012). The situation described above has accorded the country a devastating compendium among the committee of nations.

To address this challenge, this chapter argues that the huge financing gap in the water sector must be effectively bridged. From the submission of Amakom (2008), the country needs to spend a total of N262 billion per annum from 2006 to 2015 in order to meet water and sanitation needs. Howbeit, successive budgetary allocations have fallen short of this projection. Aside from funding, other issues begging for policy attention include the moral commitment of the political actors to the realization of sectoral policy guidelines, water sector planning, data generation, monitoring and evaluation, accountability and the strengthening of institutional mechanism.

Given the importance of water to human wellbeing, this work considers it appropriate to focus on the situation in Nigeria.

The work is divided into five sections. While this piece represents the first section, the second section explores the link between access to good water and human wellbeing. The third and fourth sections focus on the Nigerian water sector profile and the political imperatives respectively. Section five is the concluding reflections.

2. Water and Wellbeing: Exploring the Nexus

As empirical evidence has suggested, access to improved water sources impacts positively on human wellbeing. Before exploring the channels through which water enhances wellbeing, it is important to clarify the concept of wellbeing. The concept of wellbeing is often used interchangeably with such concepts as quality of life, welfare, health and sustainability (Murphy, 2010: 17). The concept can be approached from different perspectives. While the hedonic perspective accentuates constructs such as happiness and satisfaction with life, the eudaimonic tradition highlights positive psychological functioning and human development (Dodge et al, 2012: 223). Consumption related definitions associate wellbeing with the consumption of goods, services, and resources (King, 2007: 11). Functioning, capabilities, and agency are the core components of the capability perspective. Functioning includes the valuable activities and states that become a person's wellbeing such as a healthy body and being safe; capabilities refer to the freedom one has to do these valuable activities and reach these valuable states; and agency is the ability to pursue goals that one has reason to value (Deneulin and McGregor, 2010: 504-505). At the community level, wellbeing can be subsumed under three categories. These include sustainable development, health and quality of life, and economic-centred considerations such as gross domestic product and human development index (Murphy, 2010: 17). From the above submissions, wellbeing connotes a state of wellness, happiness, and satisfaction that impacts positively on the quality of life.

How is wellbeing achieved? Although what translates into wellbeing may differ from person to person or group to group, particularly if the concept is examined from the subjective angle, but with reference to the primary measures of wellbeing, access to basic services forms the core. These basic services include portable water, primary healthcare, education, and even electricity. If these services are out of reach, the consequence is usually deleterious. However, the delivery of good water constitutes the analytical lens here.

From primeval cultural levels to the contemporary, water has been of paramount importance to mankind. Traditional societies were able to develop technologies in order to construct wells, refurbish natural springs, devise irrigation scheme, and create elaborate methods with which to provide their populations with water (Novo, 2012: 65). Water use falls into several major classes, each of which is associated with certain quantity and quality requirements. These include water for drinking and cooking, waste disposal, crop production, aquaculture, livestock, industrial use, recreational use, navigational uses, and ecological values (Martins, 2001: 17). Rainfall and soil water are fundamental parts of all terrestrial and aquatic ecosystems which supplies goods and services for human wellbeing. Availability and quality of water determines ecosystem productivity, both for agricultural and natural systems (United Nations Environment Programme, 2009: ix). Water is a fundamental requirement for human life (Akpor and Muchie, 2011: 480) and essentially determines the overall socio-economic development of any nation (Nwankwoala, 2011: 1170). The water sector is a cross-cutting sector affecting infant mortality, maternal mortality, nutritional values, and environmental hygiene (Muta'aHellandedu, 2012: 112). Water is therefore the most important natural resource.

Water and sanitation remain the primary drivers of public health (Muta'aHellandedu, 2012: 111). Probing the health component of water, Ayoade (1975: 582) avers that the provision of pipe-borne water can help in eradicating water-borne diseases and in improving the general sanitation of towns and villages. Poor access to safe water supply has a critical health implication (Mobie and Masango, 2009: 2). The lack of access to safe water, basic sanitation and good hygiene practices is the third most significant risk factor for poor health in developing countries with high mortality rate (Sanctuary et al., 2013). It is estimated that 1.6 million deaths per year are attributed to unsafe water supply and sanitation (Haller et al., 2007:

468). The direct health benefits of improved water supply, especially when integrated with sanitation initiatives, are huge. They include safe disposal of human excreta, the use of water for hygiene purposes, and the satisfaction derived from drinking clean water (Nwankwoala, 2011: 1171). From the foregoing, the place of safe water in health management is irreducible. Water impacts greatly on human welfare by promoting better sanitary practices and preventing diseases such as dengue, diarrhoeal and high intensity intestinal helminth infections such ascariasis, trichuriasis, and hukeworm.

Again, water supply is critical to sustainable economic competitiveness of any nation (Ali, 2012). It lies at the heart of development. From the report of Sanctuary et al. (2013), improved water supply and sanitation boosts countries' economic growth and contributes greatly to poverty eradication through a number of channels: macroeconomic policies, including fiscal, monetary and trade policies, directly and indirectly affect demand and investment in water-related activities; gains from improved water supply benefit poor people most; improved water supply impacts positively on workers' health which is critical for increased production and productivity. Agriculture and food security are also critically dependent on water availability as the planting time and crop yield are both determined by the duration and amount of rainfall that is recorded in a farming season (Muta'aHellandedu, 2012: 111). Large amounts of water are used to generate the ecosystem services needed to ensure provisioning of basic supplies of food, fodder and fibers (United Nations Environment Programme, 2009: v). Food security, which is a major predictor of economic development, is guaranteed through adequate supplies of water for agricultural purposes.

The benefits derived from improved water supplies, no doubt, align with the innate attributes of wellbeing. As encapsulated by the hedonic, eudaimonic, and capability schools, improved water supply improves health and the quality of life; guarantees satisfaction with life and promotes psychological functioning, human capabilities and development.

3. Nigeria's Water Sector Profile

Providing a sustainable and improved water services to the increasing population across the developing world remains one of the biggest challenges towards meeting the water target in the millennium development goals (Addo-Yobo et al., 2006: 419). The situation in Africa is particularly devastating. Water access to 56 per cent of the African population is limited or available only from unprotected sources; several millions lack even simple improved latrines and thus exposed to different diseases; and pay a heavy toll in casualties (Novo, 2012: 66). More worrisome is the fact that the poor state of water coverage in Nigeria is worse than the situation in most African countries (Society for Water and Sanitation, 2013). Water and sanitation coverage rates in Nigeria are among the lowest in the world, and Nigeria is currently not on track to reach the MDG targets of 75 per cent coverage for safe drinking water by the year 2015 (Water and Sanitation Monitoring Platform, 2008:1). Describing the situation in Nigeria, Ayoade (1975: 588) submits that the traditional methods of water exploitation, particularly in the rural areas, consist of direct collection of rain water; and extraction from springs, streams, ponds, and wells. Water shortages during the dry season are quite common as many of these sources dry up; people then trek long distances in search of water. There is also the problem that the water is untreated and therefore carries organisms that are parasitic to man. In the assertion of Martins (2001: 22), industries in Nigerian cities rely almost entirely on independent sources of water supply for their operations due to inadequacies of government supplies. This is done through abstraction of groundwater by the construction of boreholes. As viable as this alternative may prove, it also portends danger to the environment through land subsidence, flooding and collapse of structures.

From the statistics provided by the Water and Sanitation Platform (2008: 2-3), the proportion of urban population with access to improved sources of drinking water in Nigeria decreased 15 per cent from 80 per cent in 1990 to 65 per cent in 2006. The rural areas recorded a decrease of 4 per cent from the 34 per cent in 1990 to 30 per cent in 2006. While the national access for water supply was put at 54.3 per cent in 2007, the population with access in 2008 was 58 per cent. This data implies that as many as 63 million Nigerians have no access to improved water supply (Water and Sanitation Programme, 2011: 8). The situation in Nigeria has regrettably reached a 'pressure point'. This is the point at which the existing infrastructure gets suffocated by the massive needs and demands of the populace (Oshewolo and Oniemola, 2011: 261). As a result, Nigeria has been ranked among the countries with the worst human development indicators in Africa, aside from those nations that were recently at war (IRIN, 2007). In 2012, the Food and Agricultural Organization stated during the celebration of World Water Day that 48 countries, including Nigeria, would face water shortage by 2025 (Ali, 2012). Currently, Nigeria occupies the 130th position on the Global Water Poverty index of developing countries still battling with water and sanitation accessibility (Weekly Trust, January 5, 2013).

The above state of affairs is somewhat paradoxical given the enormous potentials of Nigeria. The country is well drained with a reasonably close network of rivers and streams. There are natural water bodies like lakes as well as lagoons particularly in the coastal areas (Ayoade, 1975: 583). The Federal Ministry of Water Resources Roadmap for Nigeria's water sector estimates the water resources potential of the country as 267 and 92 billion m^3 of surface and groundwater respectively (Ali, 2012). Describing these potentials, Martins (2001) remarks that the atmospheric water Nigeria receives annually in form of rainfall is huge; the hydrospheric or surface water resources such as oceans, lakes, and rivers are enormous; and the lithospheric water in soils and rock under the soil is considerable. Nigeria's groundwater is also exploitable through springs or artificially through wells and boreholes (Ayoade 1975: 586). In view of the above reality, Nigeria has adequate surface and groundwater resources to meet current demands for portable water (Federal Republic of Nigeria, 2000: 4) if maximally exploited.

The factors responsible for the crisis in Nigeria's water sector have been identified. The capital budgets of the Ministry of Water Resources have been lamentably low. There seems to have been a deliberate and continuing curtailment of public expenditure in the sector (Oshewolo and Oniemola, 2011: 262). While the total sum of N40.94billion was spent in 2011, the sum of N43.6billion was expended in 2012 excluding the expenditures on other projects such as Goronyo Dam (N3.4billion); Kashimbila Dam (N38billion); Gurara

Dam (N36billion); Ife Dam (N3billion). In 2013, the sum of N39billion has been proposed from line budget to be spent on water related projects. This will be in addition to funds the sector will receive from special intervention funds (Jonathan, 2013). The above figures exemplify the level of government commitment to providing improved water to the citizens. Government intervention has not only been poor, it has also been responsible for the crisis in the sector. This reduction in public expenditure has precipitated a huge 'funding gap' in the sector.

According to Nwankwoala (2011: 1172), water supply has suffered from poor coordination, poor maintenance culture, poor technical institutional structure, multiple programmes, lack of data for planning, overbearing bureaucratic control by various supervising agencies, lack of professional inputs on projects, lack of community participation, inadequate funding, lack of adequate quality monitoring and evaluation. Ayoade (1975: 583) mentions inadequate planning and management of water resources; and poor distribution of water in time and space in relation to man's need. Limited civil society participation, limited human resources, irregular and conflicting statistics on sector coverage, poor sector monitoring and accountability mechanisms are other key issues (Water and Sanitation Monitoring Platform, 2008: 1). A major challenge borders on how to promulgate policy guidance at the state level as water supply is mostly the state government's responsibility. While some states have created strong enabling environments, other states are yet to start the reform process (Water and Sanitation Programme, 2011: 2). Again, the local government authorities are responsible for the provision of rural water supplies in their areas. Only a few of them have the resources and skills to address the problem. Majority of the local government areas do not have functional rural water supply divisions (Federal Republic of Nigeria, 2000: 5).

4. The Political Imperatives in Nigeria

To achieve rapid industrialization, develop as a nation and be economically competitive, it is a matter of national importance to address the problems that confront the water sector in Nigeria. Historically, a number of initiatives have been taken with a view to providing water to Nigerians. The first modern water supply scheme in the country was established in Lagos in 1915 and by 1953, 27 other waterworks had been built in various parts of the country. Only a few of these water schemes were financed by the colonial government, while the others were partially financed by the native authorities. Between 1953 and 1960, the number of towns having modern water supplies increased from 28 to 67 (Ayoade, 1975: 588). The drought of early seventies prompted the Federal Government to take a number of actions which resulted in the establishment of the Federal Ministry of Water Resources in 1976, National Water Resources Institute in 1977, and the River Basin Development Authorities in 1978 (Martins, 2001: 20). Today, all the 36 states and the Federal Capital Territory have Water Corporations or Public Utilities Boards managing their public water supply (Ali, 2012).

There have also been a number of legislations and strategy documents in the water sector. Aside from the constitution of the Federal Republic of Nigeria, there is the Water Resource Act 101 of 1993, which empowers the Federal Ministry of Water Resources to regulate, develop, and license all water operators in Nigeria, in addition to planning and usage of water resources, management of water resources and application of appropriate standards (Akpor and Muchie, 2011: 483). Other key policy documents and model laws in the water sector National Water and Sanitation Policy (2000), National Water Policy (2004), National Water Sanitation Policy (2006), National Water Resources Strategy (2006), Draft National Water Bill (Water and Sanitation Programme, 2011: 14). From the foregoing, Nigeria has never lacked water policies and initiatives. The problem has been the absence of effective coordination, monitoring and evaluation. What then are the political imperatives?

First, the various water policy guidelines must be harmonized and coordinated. This is necessary for effective implementation and to prevent the conflict that the lack of sound policy harmonization and coordination may generate. Some of the policy guidelines in these strategy documents contain ambitious plans. For instance, the National Water Supply and Sanitation Policy adopted in January 2000 made the supply of adequate water and sanitation a right of all Nigerians, and gives responsibility to the three tiers of government, the private sector, and the beneficiaries. It identifies the need for reforms and recognizes the special needs of women and the poor, and the need to link improved sanitation with water supply (Federal Republic of Nigeria, 2000: 5). What is required is the moral commitment of the political actors to the realization of these noble goals. The realization of these goals underscores the need for rational planning in the sector. Effective planning would prevent the events of flood, rural and urban water shortages that have become regular occurrences in Nigeria; help the country to leverage on its abundant water resources; and help harmonize the efforts of the three tiers of government including the private sector and non-governmental organizations. Given the uneven spatial distribution of water resources in Nigeria, an accurate assessment of the water resources of any area therefore requires knowledge of not only the magnitude of rainfall and its spatial and temporal distribution but also the nature and magnitude of rainfall of water losses by evaporation (Ayoade, 1975: 583). Howbeit, without data, how do we plan and make projections into the future? Government must, of necessity, improve on sectoral data generation and harmonization to aid effective planning.

The human factor must also be considered. Government at all levels have very limited human resources capacity for the implementation of the sector activities (Water and Sanitation Monitoring Platform, 2008: 1). Because rainfall and surface water represent major components of Nigeria's hydrological cycle, it is important to engage experts in the field in the management of the country's water sector. Appointments into sensitive offices in the sector must transcend political considerations, which have been the case in Nigeria. Again, given the fact the current budgetary allocations to the sector are very poor; government at all levels must increase investments in the water sector. Huge government investments are needed to achieve the different policy guidelines, and achieve the MDG target set for 2015. Alternative sources of funding by the private sector and development partners may also be mobilized. However, government sectoral monitoring systems must be improved upon. This will properly inform decisions on national water sector investments, sub-sector resource allocation, sub-national disbursing, accountability of funds and actual disbursement (Water and Sanitation monitoring Platform, 2008: 1). Leakages in government through official corruption must also be blocked. Corruption in government will not only drain investible funds in the water sector, it will also degrade the existing water infrastructures.

Since nothing on this earth has life without good water, drinking water standards must be enforced. Drinking water quality standards must ensure the absolute safety of all drinking water supplies to safeguard public health. To achieve this goal, institutional mechanisms must be put in place. Legislations must be passed to strengthen bodies such as the Nigerian Industrial Standards and National Agency for Food and Drug Administration and Control, among others.

5. Concluding Reflections

The role of improved water supplies in the development of human wellbeing, management of health, and transformation of the economy cannot be overemphasized. As argued in the body of this work, human functioning – health, psychological, economic – is heavily dependent on the quantity and quality of water resources available. Talking about the availability of water resources, Nigeria demonstrates a huge potential. Nigeria's water resources exist in the shapes of atmospheric, hydrospheric, lithospheric, and groundwater supplies. These resources notwithstanding, access to improved water supplies in Nigeria has been worrisomely low. This is the situation in both the urban and rural areas. This situation has also accorded Nigeria poor statistical rankings globally and continentally. Although successive governments have adopted different measures to address the problem of water shortages, but the impact has been minimal. To address the problem and promotes sustainable access to improved water supplies in Nigeria, the paper recommends the moral commitment of the political actors to water generation and distribution, effective planning, monitoring and evaluation, blockage of leakages in government through official corruption, and a significant increase in the budgetary allocation to the sector.

References

Addo-Yobo, F., Njiru, C., and Sohail, M. (2006), 'Determinants of Households' Intention to Pay for Improved Water Services: An

Application of the Theory of Reasoned Action', in *Journal of Water Supply: Research and Technology*, 55(6): 419-425.

Africa Public Health (2012), *Combined Global and African Ranking – 25 Country Populations with the Least Sustainable Access to Improved/Clean water Sources*, Available at http://www.info.who.int/pmnch/media/news/2012/201205_africa_scorecard.pdf (Accessed: 20 October 2013).

Akpor, O.B and Muchie, M. (2011), 'Challenges in Meeting the MDGs: The Nigerian Drinking Water Supply and Distribution Sector', in *Journal of Environmental Science and Technology*, 4(5): 480-489.

Ali, K.A. (2012), 'Development of Water Supply Infrastructure in Nigeria: Challenges and Prospects', Being 2012 Nigerian Society of Engineers October Lecture.

Amakom, U. (2008). *Nigeria: Effective of Local Governments to Provide Water and Sanitation Services,* A WaterAid Report, WaterAid.

Ayoade, J.O. (1975), 'Water Resources and their Development in Nigeria' in *Hydrological Sciences*, XX (4): 581-591.

Carter, J.G. (2007), 'Spatial Planning, Water and the Water Framework Directive: Insights from Theory and Practice', in *The Geographical Journal*, 173(4): 330-342.

Daily Times, NG, (2012), *Nigeria has 3rd Poorest Water Supply,* May 12, Available at: http://www.dailytimes.com.ng/article/nigeria-has-3rd-poorest-water-supply (Accessed: 20 October 2013).

Deneulin, S and McGregor, J.A. (2010), 'The Capability Approach and the Politics of a Social Conception of Wellbeing', in *European Journal of Social Theory*, 13(4): 501-519.

Dodge, R., Daly, A.P., Huyton, J. and Sanders, L.D. (2012), 'The Challenge of Defining Wellbeing', *International Journal of Wellbeing*, 2(3): 222-235.

Federal Republic of Nigeria (2000), 'Water Supply and Sanitation Interim Strategy Note', November, Abuja: Nigeria.

Haller, L., Hutton, G. and Bartram, J. (2007), 'Estimating the Costs and Health Benefits of Water and Sanitation Improvements at the Global Level', in *Journal of Water and Health*, 5(4): 467-480.

Integrated Regional Information Network (IRIN) (2007), *Nigeria: Basic Services a Challenge to Nigeria's Leaders,* IRIN, UN.

Jonathan, G. (2013), *President Jonathan's Address at the Presidential Summit on Water*, Abuja: State House. Available at: hhtp://www.statehouse.gov.ng/index.php/news/speeches/87-president-jonathan-s-address-at-the-presidential-summit-on-water (Accessed: 20 October 2013).

King, P. (2007), *The Concept of Wellbeing and its Application in a Study of Ageing in Aotearoa New Zealand,* Enhancing Wellbeing in an Ageing Society (EWAS) Working Paper Series, No. 8, New Zealand.

Martins, O. (2001), 'Water Resources Management and Development in Nigeria – Issues and Challenges in a New Millennium', An Inaugural Lecture Delivered at the University of Agriculture, Wednesday, 22 August, 2001.

Mobie, T.R. and Masango, M. (2009), 'Privatisation of Water Resources: Crime against Humanity', in *HTS Teologiese Studies/ Theological Studies*, 65(1): 1-6.

Muta'aHellandedu, J. (2012), 'Health Implications of Water Scarcity in Nigeria', in *European Scientific Journal*, 8(18): 111-117.

Murphy, B. (2010), *Community Wellbeing: An Overview of Concept*, Ontario, Canada: Nuclear Waste Management Organization (NWMO).

Novo, F.G. (2012), 'Moral Drought: The Ethics of Water Use', in *Water Policy*, 14: 65-72.

Nwankwoala, H.O. (2011), 'Localizing the Strategy for Achieving Rural Water Supply and Sanitation in Nigeria', in *African Journal of Environmental Science and Technology*, 5(13): 1170-1176.

Oshewolo, S. and Oniemola, R.M. (2011), 'The Financing Gap, Civil Society and Service Delivery in Nigeria', in *Journal of Sustainable Development in Africa*, 13(2): 254-268.

Punch (2012), '70 Million Nigerians lack Access to Portable Water – Minister', February 24, Available at http://www.punchng.com/business/business-economy/70-million-nigerians-lack-access-to-potable-water-minister/ (Accessed: 18 October 2013).

Sanctuary, M., Troop, H. and Berntell, A. (2013), *Making Water a Part of Economic Development*, World Health Organization, Available at: http://www.who.int/water_sanitation_on_health/waterandmacroeconomics/en/_ (Accessed 29 October 2013).

Society for Water and Sanitation (2013), 'Water and Sanitation: The Nigeria Situation', *Newsletter*, January – March.

United Nations Environment Programme (2009), *Rain Water Harvesting: A Lifeline for Human Wellbeing,* A Report Prepared for UNEP by Stockholm Environment Institute, Nairobi, Kenya: UNEP.

Water and Sanitation Monitoring Platform (2008), *Water and Sanitation Summary Sheet: Nigeria,* WSMP.

Water and Sanitation Programme (2011), *Water Supply and Sanitation in Nigeria: Turning finance into Services for 2015 and Beyond*, Nairobi, Kenya: WSP.

Weekly Trust (2013), *Adequate Drinking Water still a tall dream in Nigeria.* January 5, Available at: http://weeklytrust.com.ng/index.php/features/10559-adequate-drinking-water-still-a-tall-dream-in-nigeria (Accessed: 27 October 2013).

Chapter 11

Impact of Distance between On-site Sanitation and Location of Boreholes on Groundwater Contamination:

The Case of Developing and Semi-developed Rural Areas of Limpopo Province, South Africa

Matodzi M Mokoena & Murembiwa S. Mukhola

1. Introduction

South Africa is situated at the southern tip of the African continent, with varying weather conditions and yearly rainfall in its 9 provinces. It is estimated that more than 400 communities in South Africa depend on groundwater for domestic purposes; groundwater accounts for between 13% and 15% of all water used in the country (Pietersen, 2005). Groundwater is one of the natural water resources (like rivers, dams and lakes) that are regulated by the

geria, reported that the quality of most of the hand-dug wells is affected by the distance away from pollution sources, and the effect of distance was more pronounced in terms of faecal and total coliform counts, which decreased with increasing distance from waste dumps. There is a high degree of contamination from hand-dug wells during the rainy season while the wells dry up during the dry season. Machingambi and Manzungu (2003) reported that the water level in the both groundwater and surface-water sources decreases in winter while it increases in the summer. In the study that assessed the public and private boreholes in South Africa, Potgieter et al. (2006) established that during the rainy season 55% of private and 70% of communal borehole water samples tested were classified as good (0 CFU per 100 mℓ); 25% of private and 15% of communal borehole water samples were classified as marginal (1 to 10 CFU per 100 mℓ); whereas 25% of private and 15% of communal borehole water samples were classified as poor (>10 CFU per 100 mℓ). During both the dry ($p = 0.006$) and rainy seasons ($p < 0.0001$) the difference in faecal coliform contamination was significant, although during the rainy seasons the contamination was more prevalent in private borehole water samples compared to communal borehole water samples. These boreholes in the developing and semi-developed rural areas are not properly planned during the building of the houses and other structures on the properties (Xu and Beekman, 2003). Contamination of the private boreholes in developing and semi-developed rural areas as well as poor planning could become issues of concern and could be the catalysts as potential sources of groundwater contamination (Davies, 2002).

Research question

What is the effect of the distance between the privately owned boreholes and potential sources of contamination (pit latrines and animal droppings) on the faecal contamination of borehole water using *Enterococci* and *Escherichia coli* as indicators of water pollution by faecal material in developing and semi-developed rural areas in the Limpopo Province. *Escherichia coli* and *Enterococci* should be absent unless faecal contamination is present (Department of Water Affairs and Forestry, 1996).

Methodology

Study area description: Sinthumule under Makhado Municipality

This study was conducted in the northern part of South Africa, in Limpopo Province, Makhado Municipality, in the developing and semi-developed rural area of Ha-Sinthumule (see Annexure 1). The Sinthumule villages are located quite close to Makhado town, but separated by large tracts of farmland. The groundwater in this area contains high levels of salt as this region is located south of the Soutpansberg Mountain range; this results in scale build-up in pipes and even blocked water pipes. The communal water system that supplies water through the piped distribution system with communal taps in the village was not operational during the study period. All the households selected for this study were equipped with boreholes in their yards and all were fully functional during the study period. At the time of the study these households relied on the boreholes for their primary source of water supply for both drinking water and domestic purposes. It should be noted that not every household in this specific area had a borehole in the yard.

Study participants

In the Sinthumule area there are 10 villages under Chief Sinthumule; the positions of selected households in these villages were marked using the global positioning system (GPS) and their unique coordinate number was given as the household number. Out of 500 households that have boreholes in their yards, 60 households were randomly selected and requested to participate in the study. The study outline, methodology and objectives were explained to the participants and informed consent from all participants and their principals was sought.

Ethics

This study involved people and information pertaining to their households; therefore prior to commencing with the study, ethics approval from the Tshwane University of Technology Research

Committee was obtained. Chief Sinthumule and the royal councillors granted consent to work with the communities within the study area. In all participating households, informed and formal consent was obtained from the head of the household and the senior matriarch was assigned as respondent who provided the information related to the study.

Household water information collection

A closed-ended structured questionnaire was used during the interview with the members of the household. Observations around the location of water boreholes were also recorded.

Distance measurement

The position locations of the households' boreholes, pit latrines and/or septic tanks from each randomly selected household were collected by the global positioning system (GPS) as waypoints (Garmin 60 Csx®). Thereafter the coordinates were downloaded using OziExplorer® GPS Mapping Software. Distances between each of the selected source points were measured using GPS coordinates, and the straight-line distance between each of the selected households' boreholes, pit latrines and/or septic tanks was measured in metres. Of 60 households with boreholes and pit latrines, 20 households were randomly selected and the actual distances from the boreholes to their respective pit latrines and/or septic tanks were marked using GPS.

Water quality

To determine the quality of the water from the boreholes, groundwater samples were collected directly from the borehole before the water was piped to the storage tanks. This was done in all households that store water in the tanks; permission was requested before we connected the spigot to the pipe that was supplying water to the storage tanks and the water from the spigot was assumed to represent the groundwater quality. In instances where households did not have storage tanks, water samples were collected directly from the pipes after the pipe end had been thoroughly disinfected, and allowing the water to run for 2 min or more before taking a sample. The water samples were aseptically collected from taps along the water line that connects the water source and the water-storage tank and from taps coupled to the storage tank. These taps were also used by the community members who share or buy water from these households. Finally, water samples were collected either from kitchen tap(s) or from water-storage container(s), depending on whether houses were fitted with in-house tap connections or whether households were storing water in containers. Water samples were collected twice at each sampling point mentioned above, once during late summer and once in early winter. All water samples were collected and stored in cooler boxes before being transported to the laboratory where the analyses were done within 20 min. *Escherichia coli* and *Enterococci* were used as indicators of faecal pollution. For the purposes of this study good quality water should have zero number of indicator organisms (0 *E. coli* per 100 mℓ) as is acceptable in terms of both local and international drinking water standards (Department of Water Affairs and Forestry, 1996; World Health Organization, 2006).Therefore the mean numbers and percentages of organisms per sampling unit were used to represent the worst-case scenario. The Quanti-Tray® - Colilert®-18 method (IDEXX, 2001a) and the Quanti-Tray® - Enterolert® method (IDEXX, 2001b) were used to enumerate *E. coli* and *Enterococci*, respectively, according to the manufacturers' protocol.

Animal droppings

A structured questionnaire was used during the face-to-face interview with the designated member of the household to collect data about the household's background information as well as other information required for the study, such as the use of compost for crop fertilisation. The interview was followed up by observations of the yard, noting the location of animal enclosures, and assessing the spread of animal droppings, with particular focus on the faeces of animals such as cattle, goats, sheep, dogs, pigs, chickens and donkeys.

Analyses and contribution

It was found that in almost all the 20 households surveyed in developing and semi-developed rural areas as well as in the townships, the yards had not been planned properly before building the houses. All households randomly selected to participate in the study were found to have pit latrines placed in the corner of the yards, right next to those of their neighbours. GPS coordinates were successfully used to measure the straight line between the pit latrine and the borehole.

The councillors in this area have a policy that when a new home is built on newly proclaimed land, the first thing that needs to be built is a toilet structure, and failure to comply with this policy will lead to a fine of R150.00 (approximately $19.00). From a health perspective it is an important issue; however, problems could arise in future as site plans showing the proposed housing structures and location of boreholes are not always available at the time, and boreholes that are drilled at a later stage could lead to problems, as the toilet structure could be closer than desirable to the borehole in terms of the prevention of seepage. Due to municipal water-supply problems, many residents in the area drill their own boreholes for their private drinking-water supply and household water needs, Contrary to the toilet policy in the study area, there is no specific time limit for drilling a borehole; this depends on each individual and is based on whether or not he/she can afford to do so.

It was found that the existing vacant lots in the study area did not meet the minimum lot-size standards of accommodating most of the basic needs of the households in developing and semi-developed rural areas. In existing suburbs sizes with a minimum area in the extent of 1 350 m^2 and with a minimum street frontage of 30 m will be recognised in terms of the provisions in the municipal bylaw (Anonymous, 2001).

Some of the properties in the developing and semi-developed rural areas of the Ha-Sinthumule area of Makhado Municipality are 1 665 m^2 in size, which is not large enough for typical rural community members to provide them with all the space they need for their particular lifestyle, and most of the urban lots are 1 365 m^2 in size. The traditional leaders and councillors in developing and semi-developed rural areas decided to downsize the yard space due to an increase in demand for accommodation as the population increases. A traditional yard space in most developing and semi-developed rural areas in South Africa would normally comprise the following: housing structures; gardening for crops; animal shelter; and on-site sanitation. Due to the municipal water-supply constraints, the same yard space is now also used for drilling a borehole.

Distance of pit latrine vs. indicator organisms

The distance between the pit latrine and the borehole plays a major role in the faecal contamination of groundwater, even though the groundwater contamination takes place over time. In densely populated areas with many pit latrines there may be a substantial difference in the time taken for contamination of the groundwater to occur. All water samples from privately owned boreholes were analysed for Enterococci and E. coli and the results are given in Table 1; the respective distances between boreholes and pit latrines are also shown. For the purpose of this study a count of zero indicator organisms per 100 mℓ of sample was used as the standard for acceptable water quality; however, any distance of more than 20 m was assumed to be an acceptable distance between a pit latrine and a borehole to prevent faecal contamination, while the international guideline uses 25 m as an acceptable distance (Dzwairo et al., 2006). Banks et al. (2002) suggested a distance of 15 m between a borehole and a pit latrine in areas that contain highly permeable or fissured strata. The soil structure and the water movement were not the main focus of this study therefore no results are presented in this study. Numbers of *E. coli* and *Enterococci* in the borehole water samples were shown as counts per 100 mℓ for the percentage of positives in these samples.

Table 1: Comparison of distances between water boreholes and pit latrines and faecal groundwater contamination using *E. coli* and *Enterococci* as indicators of water quality

Water sources	Indicators	Statistics: Confidence interval (CI)	Distance of borehole from pit latrines					
			% number	>1 m but <20m	% number	>20 m but <30m	% number	Anything >30m
Spigot	*E. coli*	CI upper 95%	*n*7 (37%)	2	*n*5 (26%)	0.5	*n*3 (16%)	0.1
		CI lower 95%		1		0.3		0.1
	Enterococci	CI upper 95%	*n*7 (37%)	178	*n*5 (26%)	526	*n*3 (16%)	48.2
		CI lower 95%		69		175		15.3
First tap	*E. coli*	CI upper 95%	*n*6 (33%)	37	*n*5 (26%)	0.6	*n*3 (16%)	0.1
		CI lower 95%		12		0.3		0.1
	Enterococci	CI upper 95%	*n*6 (33%)	79	*n*5 (26%)	130	*n*3 (16%)	0.1
		CI lower 95%		33		52		0.1
Kitchen	*E. coli*	CI upper 95%	*n*7 (37%)	6	*n*2 (11%)	1.4	*n*3 (16%)	2
		CI lower 95%		2		0.5		0.7
	Enterococci	CI upper 95%	*n*7 (37%)	43	*n*2 (11%)	297	*n*3 (16%)	0.1
		CI lower 95%		21		94		0.1

In almost all the households surveyed no distance of less than 10 m between the boreholes and the pit latrines was observed. The water quality of privately owned boreholes in terms of distance away from the potential sources of contamination was the focus of this study. In most of the cases the actual borehole drilling sites were identified by hydrogeologists and boreholes were therefore drilled without taking into consideration the potential sources of contamination on the property.

The highly contaminated water samples from spigots (representing groundwater before being stored in the tanks) were found to be in water samples from those boreholes that were very close to the pit latrine (less than 20 m away), where the *Enterococci* counts in terms of the lower and upper limits of the 95% confidence interval ranged between 69 per 100 mℓ and 178 per 100 mℓ. *Escherichia coli* numbers were found to be as low as 1 per 100 mℓ at the lower limit of the 95% confidence interval and 2 per 100 mℓ at the upper limit of the 95% confidence interval. This might be due to the fact that *E. coli* do not survive as long as *Enterococci* under unfavourable conditions (Aydin, 2007). However, the presence of this organism in drinking water indicates the pollution of groundwater by faecal materials. There were no statistically significant differences ($p < 0.0001$) among the numbers of positives in these samples for both *E. coli* and *Enterococci* in terms of their respective distances away from the pit latrine. We also found that with increasing distances away from the pit latrine there were significant decreases in the percentage of borehole water samples contaminated by *E. coli*.

However, the findings were different for *Enterococci* counts which did not decrease with increasing distance away from the pit latrine; there was an increase in the percentage of positives in spigot water samples (175 at the lower limit of the of 95% confidence interval and 526 at the upper limit of the 95% confidence interval) taken at a distance of 20 m to 30 m between pit latrine and borehole location, compared to a distance of less than 20 m away (69 at the lower limit of the of 95% confidence interval and 178 at the upper limit of the 95% confidence interval), thereafter decreasing significantly (15.2 at the lower limit of the of 95% confidence interval and 48 at the upper limit of the 95% confidence interval) when distances between the borehole and the pit latrine increased to beyond 30 m. This might be due to the fact that the water in a borehole situated at a distance of more than 30 m away from the pit latrine takes longer to be contaminated, or the contamination does not reach the water when the borehole is placed at this distance; however, due to the ability of *Enterococci* to survive a wide variety of environmental conditions, the organisms are able to contaminate water and multiply without competition, as shown by the sampling results at the spigot. Furthermore, it has been reported that *Enterococci* show resistance under harsh conditions (Gibson et al., 2011); this is the reason why they survive for long periods of time in the groundwater even though the distance between the borehole and the pit latrine is up to 30 m away. The contamination in the kitchen water samples can be attributed to the fact that containers and/or taps used provide a favourable condition for the organisms to multiply and to the fact that re-contamination of the water may occur between the source and point-of-**use** through unwashed hands or dirty utensils. Comparing the quality of the water at the spigot and the first tap in terms of *E. coli* counts given in Table 1, it can be stated that the spigot water was less contaminated than the water of the first tap. This can be attributed to the fact that people also contaminate water as they collect it at the tap.

Animal droppings across the yard and the impact on the water quality

It was unnecessary to measure the distances between animal droppings in the yard as they were literally found to be everywhere. This study takes random distribution of animal droppings across the yard as a given. The results here are presented as the mean of the positives in water samples irrespective of whether or not there were animal droppings in the yard. The quality of the water at point sources subject to contamination by animal droppings was compared to the quality of water at point sources not subject to animal contamination. We found that 57% of the households that participated in the study kept animals on their properties and animal droppings were found scattered in their yards while 43% did not keep animals and there were no faeces around the compound. Table 2 shows the presence of the animal droppings in the yard and whether their presence impacted the quality of the groundwater. It was found that that more than 42% of spigot samples of households that have animal droppings in the yard were positive for *E. coli* (mean 0.15 per 100 mℓ) and *Enterococci* (mean 124 per 100 mℓ). Of the 43% of households without animals, 32% had positive *E. coli* counts in water samples but at a lower level (mean 1.1 per 100 mℓ) and *Enterococci* counts were lower (mean 81.9 per 100 mℓ).

Table 2: Assessing the effect of animal droppings in the yard on the quality of borehole water

Water sources	Indicators	Animal droppings in the yards			
		Yes	Organism (mean per 100 mℓ)	No.	Organism (mean per 100 mℓ)
Spigot	*E. coli*	*n*8 (42 %)	0.15	n8 (32 %)	1.1
	Enterococci	*n*8 (42 %)	124	*n*8 (32 %)	81.9
First tap	*E. coli*	*n*8 (42 %)	0.57	*n*4 (21 %)	18.8
	Enterococci	*n*8 (42 %)	52.3	*n*4 (21 %)	16.8
Kitchen	*E. coli*	*n*4 (21 %)	0.8	*n*3 (16 %)	3.1
	Enterococci	*n*3 (16 %)	2.65	*n*3 (16 %)	26.9

Escherichia coli results given in Table 2 show higher positives in water samples collected from point sources in yards without animal droppings and lower positives in yards with animal droppings. However, this is contrary to the results obtained in the *Enterococci* counts, where there were significant increases in positives in the water samples collected at point sources in yards where animals are kept compared with those without animals. This might be due to the fact that the *E. coli* was dying off due to poor environmental conditions such as drying up of the media and high temperatures in the hot sun (Bitton et al., 1983; Foppen and Schijen, 2006; Aydin, 2007). *Enterococci* have been reported as being reliable indicators of faecal contamination in groundwater, as they are able to grow and survive under harsh conditions; this might be the reason why in both instances in this study *Enterococci* successfully indicated the quality of the water (Gibson et al., 2011).

Data on the use of composted livestock and poultry manure as crop fertilisers were not reported in this study as there were not enough data to draw any firm conclusions. Distances between the boreholes and the pit latrines play a major role in the contamination of groundwater in the rural households. There was a decrease in the percentage of positives in water samples at a distance of more than 30 m between the borehole and the pit latrine in terms of both *E. coli* and *Enterococci;* however, the percentage of samples testing positive for *Enterococci* increases with increasing distances of between 1 m to less than 30 m. *Enterococci* survive as they are more environmentally resistant than *E. coli,* therefore a longer distance from the borehole does not affect the organism's ability to contaminate water. Almost all water samples collected from the boreholes that are located at a distance of less than 20 m away from pit latrines were contaminated by both indicator organisms used in this study. We did not observe any differences in the number of positives in water samples for *E. coli* related to their respective distances from pit latrines. Animal faeces contaminate the groundwater in the yards due to runoff during heavy rain events, and soil infiltration, as well as being windblown and entering pipes if these are not well protected and sealed off.

Conclusion

This study concludes that the distance between the potential contamination sources (pit latrines and animal droppings) and the location of the borehole plays a major role in leading to faecal contamination of groundwater. Statistical analyses of indicator organisms, namely *E. coli* and *Enterococci*, were used to determine faecal groundwater contamination. The use of *Enterococci* was found to be a more reliable indicator of faecal contamination in the borehole water samples tested. Even though the size of the household was not established in this study and the potential impact of contamination from the neighbour's yard on water sources was not determined, the findings of this study indicate that the average yard is not large enough to accommodate all household needs. Local government should assist households with the necessary pre-planning of the yard and a site plans. Such plans should indicating the position of all structures to be built (including the toilet structure and the housing structure) as well as garden areas, animal lairs and the location of the borehole, before any building work on the site commences. The local environmental health practitioners should monitor and control potential sources of contamination before and after drilling the boreholes and appropriate action should be taken. Drinking water obtained from privately owned boreholes needs to be constantly monitored and tested for the presence of the contaminants.

References

Adekunle, I., Adetunji, T., Gbadebo, A. and Bankjoko, O.B. (2007), 'Assessment of groundwater quality in a typical rural settlement in Southwest Nigeria', in *Environmental Research and Public Health*, 4(4): 12.

Anonymous (2001), 'Residential Zones for Communities and the Rural Area By-Law, *Discussion Paper #8.*

Aydin, A. (2007), 'The microbiological and physico-chemical quality of groundwater in West Thrace, Turkey', in *Polish Journal of Environmental Studies*, 16: 377-383.

Banks O., Karnachuk, O., Pamachev, V., Holden, W. and Frengstad, B. (2002), 'Groundwater contamination from rural pit latrines: Examples from Siberia and Kosova', in *Water and Environment Journal,* 16: 147-152.

Barnard, T., Robertson, C., Jagals, P. and Potgieter, N. (2011), 'A rapid and low-cost DNA extraction method for isolating *Escherichia coli* DNA from animal stools', in *African Journal of Biotechnology*, 10 (8): 1485-1490.

Bitton, G., Ferrah, S., Ruskin, R., Butner, J. and Chou, J. (1983), 'Survival of the pathogen and indicator organisms in ground water', in *Ground Water*, 21: 405–410.

Davies, J. (2002), *Development of a Curriculum and Training of Supervision Teams in Borehole Construction in Malawi*, Report No. CR/02/219N, British Geological Survey International Report CR.

Department of Water Affairs and Forestry (1996), *South African water quality guidelines*, Pretoria, South Africa: Department of Water Affairs and Forestry.

Department of Water Affairs and Forestry (2000), *Water Supply Service Levels*, Pretoria, South Africa: Department of Water Affairs and Forestry.

Department of Water Affairs and Forestry (2004), *Ground water protection - Involving community members in a hydrocencus*, Pretoria, South Africa: Department of Water Affairs and Forestry.

Dzwairo, B., Hoko, Z., Love, D. and Guzha, E. (2006), 'Assessment of the impacts of pit latrines on groundwater quality in rural areas: Case study from Morandera district, Zimbabwe', in *Physics and Chemistry of the Earth*, 31: 779-788.

Foppen, J. and Schijen, J. (2006), 'Evaluation of data from the literature on the transport and survival of *Escherichia coli* and thermotolerant coliforms in aquifers under saturated conditions', in *Water Research South Africa*, 40: 401-426.

Gibson, K.E., Opryszko, M.C., Schissler, J.T., Guo, Y. and Schwab, K.J. (2011), 'Evaluation of human enteric viruses in surface water and drinking water resources in Southern Ghana', in *The American Society of Tropical Medicine and Hygiene*, 84: 20-29.

IDEXX (2001a), 'Colilert®-18 An easy 18-hour test for coliforms and *E.coli*', IDEXX Laboratories, Westbrook, ME, USA.

IDEXX (2001b), 'Enterolert's an easy 24-hour test for enterococci', IDEXX Laboratories, Westbrook, ME, USA.

Machingambi, M. and Manzungu, E. (2003), 'An evaluation of rural communities' water use patterns and preparedness to manage domestic water sources in Zimbabwe', in *Physics Chemistry of the Earth*, 28: 1039-1046.

Majuru, B. (2010), *Assessing the Value of Upgrading Rural Small Community Water Supplies in Limpopo, South Africa.* MTech, Unpublished Dissertation, Pretoria, South Africa: Tshwane University of Technology.

Majuru, B., Mokoena, M.M., Jagals, P. and Hunter, P.R. (2010), 'Health impact of small-community water supply reliability', in *Intinternational Journal of Hygiene and Environmental Health*, 5: 1-5.

Mokoena, M. and Jagals, P. (2010), 'The effect of water-supply service delivery on the risk of infection posed by water in household containers', *Paper presented at the WISA 2010 International Biennial Conference*, Durban, South Africa, April 18 to 22, 2010.

Pietersen, K. (2005), 'Groundwater crucial for rural development', *Paper presented at the Biennial Groundwater Conference*, Pretoria, South Africa, March/April 2005.

Potgieter, N, Koekemoer, R, Jagals, P. (2007), 'A pilot assessment of water, sanitation, hygiene and home-based care services for people living with HIV/AIDS in rural and peri-urban communities in South Africa', in *Water Science and Technology,* 56(5): 125-131.

Potgieter, N., Mudau, L. and Maluleke, F. (2006), 'The microbiological quality of private and communal boreholes in the Tshitale-Hlanganani region of the Limpopo Province, South Africa', in *Water Science and Technology,* 54(11-12): 371-377.

Republic of South Africa (1997), *Water Services Act* (Act No. 108 of 1997). Available at: http://*www.dwaf.gov.za/Documents/Legislature/a108-97.pdf* (Accessed: 12 May 2012).

Republic of South Africa (1998), *National Water Act* (Act No. 36 of 1998). Available at: http://*www.info.gov.za/view/Download* (Accessed: 26 March 2012).

Rietveld, L. C., Haarhoff, J. and Jagals, P. (2008), 'A tool for technical assessment of rural water supply systems in South Africa', in *Journal of Physics and Chemistry of the Earth*, 34: 43-49.

United Nations (2005), *The Millennium Development Goals Report*, New York. Available at: http://www.un.org/millenniumgoals (Accessed: 01 June 2010).

Vhembe District Municipality (2009/2010), *Integrated Development Plan (IDP) Review*, Thohoyandou, South Africa: Vhembe District Municipality.

World Health Organization (WHO) (2006), *Guidelines for Drinking-Water Quality*, Geneva, Switzerland: WHO.

Xu, Y. and Beekman, H. (2003), *Groundwater Recharge Estimation in Southern Africa*, Paris: UNESCO.

Acknowledgements

We would like to extend our gratitude to the people of Ha-Sinthumule who participated in this survey. Financial support from the National Research Foundation and the Tshwane University of Technology is herewith gratefully acknowledged. We also acknowledge the valuable assistance by Mji A.

Chapter 12

Analysis of policy implication on water service indicators and basic household water service delivery in rural areas of South Africa: A Review

Lutendo S. Mudau, Murembiwa S. Mukhola & Paul R. Hunter

Introduction

Although it is the right for every human being to access water supply which is sustainable, affordable and safe (United Nations, 2013a); 760million people worldwide are still living without potable water (WHO/UNICEF, 2012). The United Nations' Millennium Development Goal (MDG) requires every country to half the number of people without access to water and sanitation by 2015 (United Nations, 2013a). Currently more than 50% of the countries worldwide have reached the target though Sub-Saharan countries are still at 47% (WHO/UNICEF, 2012). Nevertheless, South Africa (SA) is counted among those countries who reached the target by providing 93% of its communities with access to water service (WHO/UNICEF, 2012).

Despite this achievement, the disparities of water access and availability between urban and rural communities are still a formidable challenge (Water Research Commission., 2012) . Worldwide, urban areas tend to have more sustainable water supply than in rural areas (United Nations, 2013a). Since the beginning of MDG; the poor were known to be the one who suffer and was associated with unsafe water supply. It is one of the reasons why most of the rural communities spend much time collecting water far away from their household; while most of those living in urban areas enjoy benefits of having taps within their yards (Boone et al., 2011). People living in urban areas are often provided with acceptable water services while rural and informal settlements have low access to water services (Hosking and Jacoby, 2013). Provision of water services in these areas are prioritized compared to rural areas due to its economic well-being. Most rural and informal settlement communities do not enjoy such privileges because where taps are provided; frequent water supply remains a big challenge.

United Nation human rights encourage each country to develop policies that addresses water supply services provided to all (United Nations., 2013b). The SA government has realized such rights long before as indicated in the constitution stating the right to safe water supply as a mandate for each local Municipality to provide such services (SA Constitution Act 108., 1996, SA Water Service Act 108., 1997). The water and sanitation policy from the Department of Water Affairs [DWA], (1994) explains how water service should be provided. It is stated in this policy, that any water service rendered should be accessible, available and potable (Department of Water Affairs., 1994). These three concepts are regarded as the main conceptual framework to measure the level of basic water service delivery in each WSA in SA. Indicators of these concepts clearly show that 25 litre (L) of water should be available daily to every individual within 200 metre (m) at a flow rate of 10L per minute. To enhance affordability, free basic water regulation was set based on these indicators (Department of Water Affairs., 2002). The first 6000L is provided free of charge to the poor; and that was calculated using household with 8 members who should receive 25L/c/d (Litres per capita per day) in 30 days (Department of Water Affairs., 2002). The measurement was set based on quantity of water that needs to be accessed by each member of the households per day as a basic water service level required. Where such indicators are not met water service delivery service is taken as being compromised. Unfortunately most of WSA's in SA do not meet such requirements (Smith, 2010).

Currently there is no methodology that is used in SA to quantify access to basic water services provided by WSA's as benchmarked by these indicators; especially in a small localized rural areas. It is the purpose of this review to come up with a rapid methodology to estimate and quantify water accessed by a community in a village, local Municipality or WSA's; and benchmarked against the indicators that measures basic water service delivery and the risks that could be associated with it. Where adequate water supply cannot be maintained, water safety plans at household level should be employed; supported by continuous education to the affected communities. The main question will be how the WSA's could quantify risks using indicators as a way of measuring its own service delivery in rural communities?

Conceptual framework of basic water service delivery

Key issue in measuring basic water service delivery in SA; is to access continuous water supply in households without attaining any risks. To meet such requirements the water service should be available (water quantity), accessible (distance travelled and time) and potable (microbial water quality). Once these requirements are met community risks become minimal. The use of these concepts to measure basic water service delivery was made to WSA's to measure its performance when infrastructure is provided (Smith, 2010). This could assist in rating the water service delivery efficiency, effectiveness and its sustainability. Detailed analysis of each concept is discussed.

Accessibility

Howard& Bartram (2003) describe accessibility of water service as the time spent to travel and arrive at the water source; and bringing safe potable water back to the household. However they further indicated that every household should have access of 20L volume of water within a range of 1km distance in 30minutes. The 1km radius is observed as unacceptable by other authors due to the time spent which is likely more than 30 minutes as it could be influenced by many factors such as the route used , queuing time and well-being of the person collecting water (Mansour, 2011). This international standard does not include the flow rate as its standard is not limited to only one system used as compared to SA. Dar and Khan (2011) outlined some of the gaps related to the indicator as it does not consider the route used, the queuing time as well as the system used to access the water(Dar and Khan, 2011). Based on the analysis the study indicated the need for indicator's review so that it can fully inform the decision makers.

SA based its policy standard on tap water (Department of Water Affairs., 1994). This policy outlined basic water delivery as the access of 25L of water within 200m; while the average time related to this indicator is not specified as in the case with international standard. The review done by Wang & Hunter (2010) indicated that the environmental impact caused by the long distance to access water is not clear but there might be the probability of risk factors associated to that, which will require more studies to confirm the statement (Wang and Hunter, 2010).

SA is one of the countries with highest achievement in terms of MDG level on providing its communities with access to safe water when compared to other African countries. The infrastructure coverage was reported to be 97%; though the figure itself does not reflect the true reflection of sustainable basic water services (Department of Water Affairs., 2010,). Despite high infrastructure coverage; (Hay et al., 2012) indicated that many rural households have difficulties in accessing sufficient volumes of potable water in areas that is within the "served" communities due to poor maintenance; increased population leading to high water demand; leaving the communities without water for days. The incapacity of WSA'S in managing maintenance of water infrastructure remains a big challenge in SA (Hosking and Jacoby, 2013). The current water supply unrests due to water scarcity are a way of expressing dissatisfaction by the communities without access to sustainable safe water supply (Tapela, 2012).

SA water and Sanitation policy states that if water is not available, WSA's should provide the community with an alternative source within 24hrs. Most often the alternative source is not provided; leaving the community without water for months rendering the infrastructure provided inefficient (Hunter et al., 2009a). The situation often causes desperation that leads the communities to resort to unsafe water sources for the sake of survival (Tapela, 2012).

Communities will need household water safety strategies to protect themselves from risks regardless the manner in which they access their water. The distance where water is accessed determine the volume of water that the household could use; and could also determine the risks of the people living in the household as the water quantity could adversely affect its use (Pickering and Davis, 2012).

Availability

The concept, water availability refers to any system or source that is capable of producing a certain volume of safe water that could be accessed by the community at any time. Various standards were set to make the concept measurable by the users. The concept was also set internationally and most countries follow this indicators as a way of measuring its basic water availability (Howard and Bartram, 2003). SA has set its own standard based on the acceptable volume of water suitable for its communities as well as the time spent to access such volumes which together have direct impact to the management of water at home. The water quantity accessed is one of the fundamental criterions that characterize the state of water service received by the community. Where the infrastructure is accessible but water is not available; it causes confusion to the community. An alternative way of frequently monitoring the compliance of the service rendered is needed for proper intervention and prevention of risks to the community due to high number of people without water access.

Availability of potable water at home could play an important role in decreasing the household risks (Mellor et al., 2012). Jagals (2006) describes the concept, water availability as enough volume of water to the user that is potable, equitable and consistently available for the purpose of drinking and all domestic activities in a household (Jagals, 2006) ; while Sphere project (2004) define the availability of water in terms of emergency as water that do not take more than three minutes to fill a volume of 20L (Sphere Project., 2004). It is again elaborated that water should also be consistently available on regular basis, and 15L of water should be available per person per day and queuing time should not exceed more than 15 minutes. The understanding of this concept by Howard and Bartram (2003) further indicated that a minimum of 7.5L of water per person per day is enough for any person in any condition; hence this figure need further investigation to align it with specific risk level. The consistency on the availability of water is shown as the major variable in this concept that determines the level of water service within the community. However, this concept on availability needs further analysis in terms of the community water service limitation and access to this valuable resource. However, the policy governing the access of such volume of water and the time spent as well as its impact to household water availability might need further analysis in terms of the concept.

Water and sanitation policy (1994) describe water availability as the continuous supply of water on regular bases without cut-off (DWAF, 1994). The policy further explains that availability of water should not be interrupted for more than 48 consecutive hours and the local authority should take reasonable steps in providing the community with other alternative source within 24 hours. In case where water is not available at all at least 10L of water per person per day should be made available (Department of Water Affairs., 2010). The 10L water could mean acceptable water volume that could be enough for any conditions as compared to 7.5 L of water limit outlined by Howard and Bartram (2003).

Nevertheless; most WSA's in SA do not conform to these indicators. The community unrests around SA are typically influenced by shortage of water and lack of communication on basic water service delivery (Tapela, 2012, Hay et al., 2012). Poor management, lack of capacity in WSA's to ensure continuous water availability is one of the main challenge (Hosking and Jacoby, 2013) . International and SA water indicators differs; as SA do not have queuing rate that could have a major impact on the acceptable time spent for water collection. There are limited studies that made analysis of 200m radius, time spent at the collection point plus time spent to arrive at home. If the accessibility and quantity of water cannot be measured then it could be difficult to manage water service delivery.

The above standard is still a dream and a challenge to most rural areas of SA as provision of safe water is still not up to the required standard as outlined above. The recent study conducted by Majuru et al. (2012) in SA, indicated that most households do not have access to acceptable volume of water due to water cut-offs that take up to 3 months. It further indicated that the furthest one-way distance travelled to a tap is 268m while alternative sources increase the distance to 600m. Most of these households members resort to unprotected water sources (Majuru et al., 2012); while others buy from private supply (Department of Water Affairs., 2010, Evans et al., 2013), subsequently leading to an increased health risks and poverty in communities.

The availability of water in communities goes along with the provision of infrastructure and the volume of water needed for domestic purposes which is also dependent on the distance travelled, reliability of water source as well as total time spent on collection to reach the household (WHO/UNICEF, 2008). Most communities consider it most important to have continuous water services on daily basis (Bradley and Bartram, 2013). The study conducted by Hope (2006) indicated that most household are not satisfied by collecting water outside their compound as it is difficult to acquire the volume of water required (Hope, 2006) . The outcomes of the study recommend the change in policy in terms of household water supply.

It is therefore important for this study to come up with the estimate of water quantity available at the tap to determine the volume of water that could be accessed by each person in the household based on the indicators provided; versus the number of taps available in order to measure the risk or performance by the Municipalities in rendering safe water to the public. This estimate measurement will only apply in villages where taps are provided outside the household and population is known. The quality of water is also very much important when this method is used. When access to sustainable water service is not attainable, continuous communication on health risks and water treatment to ensure water safety use by the community is essential.

Potability

Availability and accessibility plays an important role in household water delivery but failing to maintain its quality could be fatal to the community served. It is a requirement for every Local Authority to ensure every drop of water supplied is safe for human consumption. Any absence of water availability and long distance travelled to collect water could become a challenge in maintaining its microbiological quality due to less quantity of water that could be acquired (Hope, 2006); which could lead to unsafe sources used (Nnaji et al., 2013). It could need the community to acquire skills to manage and treat its water used for various household activities. The more water is closer, available and accessible to the point of use the less risks (Wang and Hunter, 2010, Prüss-Üstün et al., 2008).

However, availability and accessibility should be supported by ensuring that safe water is always provided. Poor access to safe water could put the communities at risk as they usually find their alternative way of getting access to water with limited consideration on its safety. Benchmarks for both international and SA are available to measure the microbiological risks in water quality.

WHO and South African National Standard (SANS) 241 of (2006) described the potability of water as safe or drinking water that do not contain *Escherichia. coli (E.coli)* (WHO., 2008; South African Bereau of Standard, 2006). *E. coli* is one of the indicators that are used to determine water quality and the presence of faecal pollution from warm-blooded animal (WHO., 2008). Enterococcus is also one of the microbial indicators that are regarded as the better marker than *E.coli* in certain conditions (Risebro et al., 2012). It survives longer in water than *E. coli* and is found in the environment and in faecal matter(Atusinguza and Egbuna, 2012; WHO., 2008). It is recommended as the best parameter to measure health risks (Risebro et al., 2012). Both international and SA standard indicated the microbial water quality risks of these bacteria as outlined in Table 3.

In rural households, factors that contribute to household water contaminations are influenced by poor environmental conditions that include poor disposal of waste, unsanitary and inadequate protected containers, contaminated hands and dippers that disperse water, inadequate clean water vessels and containers; and poor protection against contamination due to household water behavioural practices (Sobsey, 2002; Tambekar et al., 2008). Such poor practices may contribute to poor water quality in the domestic setting. Access to safe water volume of 5OL/c/d or more per could reduce significance risk level (Moriarty et al., 2010).

The South African government regards water supplies as an essential service and also provides this as a constitutional right for its citizen to have access to clean and wholesome water (SA Constitution Act 108., 1996). The Government has placed water supplies as a priority for its citizens and strive to ensure regular safe water supply for its people. This is supported by the department of Water Affairs spending millions of rand each year on infrastructure to supply drinking water in various communities (Department of Water Affairs., 2010,). Unfortunately scarcity of water and inefficient personnel combined with poor management or incapacity of WSA's causes the systems to be unreliable (Tapela, 2012). Communities are usually left without potable drinking water for longer periods and as a result communities look for alternative sources of which most of them are often not safe for human consumption (Peter, 2010). It was also highlighted as a gap that needs to be looked at when monitoring of water services is done globally(United Nations., 2013). This renders the water service provided by the Municipality ineffective (Hunter et al., 2009b). Unfortunately these conditions make poor households to resort to unprotected sources and become more vulnerable to risks.

Nevertheless provision of potable water by the WSA's does not guarantee the safety of water when it reaches the household (Künzle and Morgenroth, 2011). That could only depend on the quality of water accessed by the community at the point of collection to the point of use (Mokoena and Jagals, 2009). However application household water safety precautions are essential to prevent risks.

Household water safety and management

Water Safety Plan (WSP) model is the only acceptable criterion that is currently used and recommended by various countries to mitigate the risks in water, by implementing best practices to ensure continuous supply of safe water from the source to the consumer (Hunter et al., 2010; Bartram, 2009). Almost every region in the world today including SA have implemented the WSP; and the main reason being to

> *manage and control the activities within the water chain system; implement and identify the opportunities for low cost improvements on operation practices that enhance water safety; prevent water deterioration during distribution, handling and storage in households; improve the stakeholder communications and collaboration within water sector and give understanding to water users on complete water chain and its vulnerability* (Gelting, 2009).

However, monitoring of risks at household level in poor and rural households is limited; though sustainable water service delivery and provision of water that is safe could not be guaranteed in most developing countries (Clasen, 2010; Evans et al., 2013).

The Blue Drop certification strategy introduced through incentive-based regulation on 11th September 2008; is one of drinking water strategy that is used in SA to monitor the compliance of drinking water systems to its WSA's (Department of Water Affairs., 2009). The purpose of this regulation is to manage risks by providing the quality of water from point of generation to the tap water on the street, in household yard with or without the meter. The regulation indicates government commitment in providing safe potable water to its communities (Department of Water Affairs., 2010). It is unlikely that the focus dwell much at the tap and not extended to the point of use. The mitigation of risks given to these communities is not consistent and it dwells much at the water source to the tap on the street or yard hence it is well proven that there is a challenge of water quality access and deterioration in the household at the point of use which render the treatment at the source less efficient (Taulo et al., 2008). This may well indicates the need for managing potable water from the source to a household level and at the point of use to improve quality of life. Due to water scarcity in some rural and informal settlements of SA, there is a need for a country to shift its focus from the street tap to the household by encouraging good water practices at the domestic level.

SANS 241 and quality of domestic water supplies are used as recommended standard for water quality (South African Bureau of Standard., 2006; Department of Water Affairs., 1998). The system assessment in the WSP is to identify events that have ability to make potable water harmful and no longer fit for human consumption within the water supply chain system comparing them with standard. If hazards are identified, it informs stakeholders that the water is not potable and will become more dangerous than its original state (WHO, 2011). It is expected that such analyses should prompt the stakeholders to inform the community members to take reasonable steps to ensure the water they use is safe. In case where communities contribute to some of the hazards and mitigation steps to reduce such risks are known; they could be encouraged to stop or to become part of the solution by taking reasonable steps such as water treatment to prevent further impact of risks. Monitoring the water sources or the supply chain system is the most important step that is aimed at identifying the risks that might occur in the water source making it unsafe and not suitable for human consumption (Davison et al., 2005).

Determination of risks in an area is usually determined by the accessibility, availability and water quality. When water is not accessible and available, it will be difficult to implement the WSP. The situation could be more of challenge when the households had to find drinking water somewhere or in unprotected sources other than the one obtained from protected sources provided by the WSA. The location in which water used for drinking is found plays a crucial role in water safety. Where community access water from different sources, it becomes complicated to determine the way in which risks could be identified; and WSP approach could change following the situation in which communities find themselves. The availability of policies and strategic document could assist in assessing and measurement of basic water service delivery for effective compliance to the standard set.

Policies and documents regulating basic water service delivery in South Africa.

Policy is described as one of deliberate tools aiming to address various issues or challenges that need an action within an institution or sector so that proper resources could be adequately allocated (De Coning and Sherwill, 2004). United Nations (UN) requires every country to develop policy or strategy that ensures the provision of safe potable water that is accessible, available, acceptable and potable to its people (United Nations., 2013b). Where safe water cannot be provided sustainably; precautionary measures need to be taken.

Access to safe water is the fundamental human right and paying attention to these rights to ensure the beneficiaries be part of the issues that affect them through access to information is essential; to understand and act in a rightful way (Sphere Project., 2004). To ensure that the right to water is met, SA has developed a policy that provide free basic water to poor (Department of Water Affairs., 2002). To scale up access to safe water household water safety policy was recommended and a target of 30 countries with this policy is expected to be reached by 2015 (WHO/UNICEF, 2012). It was emphasized that the development of the policy should not hinder the main objective of providing continuous water service to the community; but should be taken as a way of ensuring sustainable safe water use.

Most of these countries emphasize the provision of safe water as a critical strategy in eradicating poverty and improving the status of health. However most of the policies in these countries recommended that, every water supply project or programme should follow reasonable measures that will aid in preventing risks in water (United Nations, 2013a; Wate, 2012). The slow pace in the implementation of such policies could cause more risks to the community.

South African Constitution Act no 108 of (1996) emphasizes the rights of every citizen in SA to have access to basic potable water supply(SA Constitution Act 108., 1996). The WSA's should ensure that these rights are met by providing water to its communities as outlined by Water Service Act no 108 of (1997)(SA Water Service Act 108., 1997). The implementation of these legislations is outlined within the framework of SA Water and Sanitation policy of (1994). The policy demonstrates the importance of safe water access and availability at all times. In terms of how water services should be delivered; SA has developed strategies, policies and legislations addressing water service delivery as shown in Table1.

Table 1: Strategic documents and legislations on basic water service delivery in South Africa

Policy/ legislation	Main Theme	Key issues addressed	Reference
National water supply and Sanitation Policy	Provision of safe water to the community	Access, affordable, availability and provision of potable water.	(Department of Water Affairs., 1994)
SA Constitution Act (108 of 1996)	Bill of rights	Right to safe water	(SA Constitution Act 108., 1996)
Water Service Act (108 of 1997)	Provision of water service by WSA's	Water service in relation to drinking water provided by the Municipalities.	(SA Water Service Act 108., 1997)
National Water Act (36 of 1998)	Water Regulation	Water regulation in relation to protection, use, management, conservation and control.	(National Water Act., 1998)
Municipal Structures Act (117 of 1998)	Powers and functions of District Municipalities	Water, sanitation and Municipal functions aiming at prevention of communicable diseases.	(Municipal Structures Act., 1997)
Free basic water implementation strategy	free basic water service regulation	Free basic water provided to the poor	(Department of Water Affairs., 2002)
Drinking water regulation strategy	Provision of safe water	Monitor, manage, communicate on water service delivery and regulate water quality.	(Department of Water Affairs., 2005)

SA drinking water quality management performance "Blue Drop".	Sustainable provision of safe water by WSA's.	WSA adhere to safe water standard SANS 241 to ensure provision of safe water to the community	(Department of Water Affairs., 2009)
National Water Services Regulation Strategy	Regulating national water services	Protecting the interest of the consumer and public through effective regulation of water supply and sanitation services	(Department of Water Affairs., 2010)

Table 2: Comparative analysis of basic water access and availability between international and South African standard

International water accessibility indicators				**Universal description**	**SA water accessibility indicators**		
Water Service level	**Distance and time spent on water collection**	**Water volume available per capita per day**	**References**	**Description of Household water service outcomes(SA and international indicators)**	**One-way water collection distance and time spent.**	**Estimate water volume available per person in the household**	**References**
Bad water service delivery	>1000m >3o min	<7.5L-15L/c/d	(Bartram and Howard, 2003; Sphere project, 2004)	Risk of utilizing unsafe water sources	>200m time not specified	<10L/p/d	DWA, 2010
Acceptable basic water service	≤1000m ≤30 min	20L/c/d	Bartram and Howard (2003)	Acceptable basic household water required with minimal risk.	<200m time not specified	25L/p/d	DWA, 1994
good water service for all	Household water connection available in the yard.	50-60L/c/d	Bartram and Howard (2003)	Preferred household water that each person should access daily - low risk	50L/c/d	50L/c/ d	DWA, 2010
Excellent water service	More than one water connection within the household	100-300L/c/d	Howard and Bartram, 2003; Moriatry et.al, 2011	Outstanding household water service delivery with very low risk.	Not specified	Not specified	None

Table 3: Water quality indicators based on both international (WHO, 2008) and SA Standard (South African Bureau of Standard, 2006; Department of Water Affairs, 1998)

		SA water quality standard					International Standard				
Determinant	Units	No risk	Low risk	Medium	High risk	Very high risk	No risk	Low risk	Medium	High risk	Very high risk
pH	at 25°C	5-6	6-9	9-9.5	9,5-10	>10	6.5	>6.5-8.5	9.-9.5	No standard	No standard
Conductivity	Mg/L at 25°C	<70	70-150	150-370	370-520	>520	<47	48-93	94-140	141-187	>187
Turbidity	NTU	<0.1	0.1-1	1-20	20-50	>50	<1	1-5	No standard	No standard	No standard
Total Coliform	CFU/100mL	<1	1-10	>10-100	>100-1000	>1000	<1	1-10	11-100	101-1000	>1000
E-Coli	CFU/100mL	<1	1	>1-10	11-100	>100	<1	1-10	11-100	101-1000	>1000
Enterococci	CFU/100mL	<	1	>1-10	11-100	>100	<1	1-10	11-100	101-1000	>1000

Table 1 indicate some of the legislations and strategic documents in SA that address access to water service. The Municipal Structures Act (117 0f 1998) establishment of WSA'S to be responsible for water issues in the Municipality; while Water Service Act (107 of 1998) indicates that it should ensure that the service is given without failure. Unfortunately the basic water indicators are not taken into consideration when such service is rendered. Table 2 indicates the water service level and its association with risk of using unsafe water sources or less quantity of water that could have impact on public health. However Table 3 shows the quantitative measurement of physical and microbiological parameters that will have health risks on human beings when consuming unsafe water. This study argues that the water service level indicators that are recommended do not cover all the factors that are needed to make measure the effectiveness of the service. Apparently the WSA's in rural areas could not measure its service using such indicators. However it is emphasized that only good quality water should be used. The study found that there is a need for WSA's to measure its service level especially in rural areas where taps are provided without meters and the sustainability of water service is a challenge. The following methodology is recommended.

Estimate measurement for basic water service delivery using conceptual framework indicators

Prior to 1994 democracy there was no measurable indicator that governs the level of basic water service delivery in SA. The right of everyone to have access to safe water was first defined by African National Congress (ANC) in Reconstruction and development Programme (RDP) of 1994 (African National Congress., 1994). That was followed by white paper Policy developed in November 1994. It is from this paper where indicators for basic water service delivery were defined in terms of accessibility availability and potability. In 1996, a Constitution was developed which emphasized the right to clean water services to all (SA Constitution Act 108., 1996). More policies and legislations were developed aiming on the improvement of basic water and sanitation services.

Starting from 1994 to 2004 a total of 13.4million people were provided with basic water supply through various government structures while further 10 Million were provided through the Department of Water Affairs (DWA). The current challenge is that not all taps provided especially in rural areas; could produce enough volume of water for each person (DWA, 2010). To determine the WSA's performance on water services; we have developed an estimate measurement of household water availability per capita per day equation in terms of indicators outlined in water and sanitation policy of 1994 and DWA (2010). Indicators were further broken down according to scores that quantity level of basic water service delivery assessment by WSA's as shown in Tables 4, 5 & 6.

Monitoring of water services done by WHO and UNICEF (2012) is measured through the population census based on the infrastructure provided; counting figures of improved and non-improved facilities used (WHO/UNICEF, 2012). The challenge with this method is that it does not consider the sustainability of basic water supply and water quality issues. The other difference is that their survey is done on a larger scale rather than in localized area. Though it is known that the sustainability of water services is crucial when such surveys are done, there is no accurate information given on reliability of the services rendered. Mansour (2011) developed a way of measuring water accessibility and availability by using GIS (Mansour, 2011). The uniqueness of this method is that it is one of the methods that could be used in a small localized area but need a technical skill to apply it. Water Aid has developed its own methodology which is an accurate way of measuring water accessibility using Global point System (GPS) to count the functionality and non-functionality of systems used within the area of service (Water Aid., 2009). The disadvantage of this method is that it takes long and it needs financial resources to be executed.

The methodology that proposed is a rapid estimation of measuring quantity of water that is available for each person against the number of systems available as well as its functionality. Taps for other use other than household activities should be excluded. The advantage of using this method is that, it does not need a specialized skill but anyone who can do a simple counting could easily use it as long as correct figures and records are available. It is fast and could give a clear indication on the actual volume of water accessed by community at that time. Its limitation is that, it is not accurate; though it can give reflection on the kind of service that people receive. Hence it can also alert the WSA'S on the risks that could be faced by the community as outlined on the service delivery ladder framework outlined by (Moriarty et al., 2010). The main reason for using this methodology is to measure systems effectiveness in delivering the quantity of water required for each person in the household. This method is similar to the one on equitable access score-card as outlined by UN (2013) as it requires self-assessment using water service indicators (United Nations., 2013b). The only difference is that it uses combination of scores with equations as outlined below.

Availability assessment

Methodology for rapid estimate measurement for availability, accessibility and potability of water service delivery in household found in small localized area is explained as follows

Availability

$$Availability = \frac{\frac{Vol}{h} \times \frac{h}{day} \times No.functional\ taps}{Population\ size}$$

To determine the volume of water that could be accessed by each person in the household; the following formula was developed:
Total number of functional taps (taps with running water) versus non-functional.

- Total number of population(count total number of households and multiply by average number of people as per census results)
- Total number of hours per day when water is available (count number of hours when water is available)
- Volumes of water that could be accessed in an hour (measure the tap up and low slope; and the one in the middle. Open the tap to its full, count litres of water that can be accessed in a minute; multiply that by 60 minutes then you will get volume of water per hour. Add each volume of water per hour and divide it by 3 then you can get an average volume per hour of the entire village.)

The equation determines the average litres of water that could be accessed by each person in a household. The results could be measured against the risks as outlined in Table 4 and by Howard and Bartram (2003) as outline in Table 2. Intervention measures could be employed based on the outcomes. The methods suggest that having water each day at different intervals or provided at a low pressure does not mean that the WSA's are conforming to the standard. Especially in areas where water cannot be provided continuously but scheduled intervals are used. The availability of water and its risks below were calculated in terms of (1994) water and sanitation policy.

Table 4: availability scores

Risk level	No of days water unavailable
No threat	Water available 24hours
Tolerable	Water not available for various days within a year
Peripheral	Water not available for a week
Not tolerable	Water not available for more than a week –not sequence

The above score were done in terms of water availability. Where water is not available for the whole week is considered medium but could be a threat to the immune compromised individuals; if water is not available more than a more , WSA's should intervene by delivering water education or water to the communities to prevent health risks. Studies done by Majuru et al. (2010) showed the increase in number of acute diarrhoea linked to major disturbances in water service; while Howard and Bartram (2003) link the volume of water accessed with the level of service (Howard and Bartram, 2003). The outcomes of water quantity outlined in water availability equation could be benchmarked with the level of service as outlined in Table 2 based on the large spectrum done by Howard and Batram, 2003; DWA, 2004; DWA, 2010).

Accessibility assessment

To determine the water accessibility in terms of distance travelled the following equation was also developed:

Accessibility= Proportion of population travelling ≤200m to collect water:

Proportion of population travelling>200 m (N≤200m: N>200m)

Table 5: Accessibility score

Risk level	Distance travelled to the tap	Position where tap is found and time interval
No threat	0-10m	Tap available in or attached to the house and access within 3minutes
Tolerable	>10-50m	Tap available within the yard access within 6 minutes
Peripheral	*>50m-200m*	Tap available on the street access within 15 minutes
Not tolerable	*>200m*	Tap on the street; unsafe sources could be used where access time is more than 20minutes

Number of household without water access within 200m should be recorded; to determine number of people who are at risk of utilizing other sources of water. According to the study done in few villages it requires up to 268m for household members to access the nearest tap which measures only the one-way trip; in areas where basic water services are provided (Department of Water Affairs., 1994). The time that a person needs to travel to the tap is not determined. If we follow the distance of 1000m roundup trip travelled in 30 minutes as determined internationally, South Africans will need 6 minutes to travel to the water point within 200m which will not always be feasible when looking at the elements that determine the route to the water point considering mountainous, round-up route, waiting periods and environmental conditions could prevent increase time to reach the water collection point. The distance of 200m need to be reviewed as it is the one way distance that does not consider the type of route used, its safety, distance travelled to come back home, mountainous or easy access route as well as total time used as outlined by Dar and Khan (2011). Crow et al. (2012) indicated that there is significance difference between the distances travelled to the source and waiting period, therefore both times need to be considered when the average water collection time if determined. The standard distance outlined in SA is quiet reasonable as compared to the international standard; though not realistic as the total time used for water fetching is not indicated.

The equation on accessibility gives an idea on the proportion of household that could walk greater than 200m and tempted to use the unimproved sources that are convenience from where they stay as indicated in Table 4. It indicated the water distances that the WSA's could determine their level of service delivery distance of 10m to 200m are considered tolerable and peripheral while distance of more than 200m considered not tolerable; placing the communities to consider using unsafe sources to their convenience. Where distance of greater than 200m is recorded, the WSA's should intervene by ensuring that safe water is brought nearer or invest in education on safe water treatment and storage. Studies confirmed that communities travel long distance to fetch drinking water but use any water that is in proximity to them for other domestic chores (Peter, 2010). This is because when water is not available, the distance to access drinking water increased making it difficult for them to access enough water required to use (Taulo et al., 2008).

Potability Assessment

The potability of water is measured according to the following scores of microbial risks that need to be benchmarked with the risk outlined on the table in terms of microbial water quality risks. WHO, (2008) measured the risk in relation to 1-5 score determining various risks, while DWA 1996 and SANS, 2006 determine the risk in terms of score 1-4. Table 4 indicated the microbial risk determined in scores 1- 4 using the risk level of good, tolerable, peripheral and not tolerable depending on the number of *E. coli* or enterococci detected per 100ml of samples. The probability of risks in terms of microbial water quality on this measurement will be rated in terms of small localised area based on dry and wet seasons due to variation of microbial activities that could occur. Previous microbiological water quality outcomes detected within a year could be used to measure the probability of risks. Where no record is available, set of samples could be taken to measure the quality of water used.

Table 4: Potability Score

Score	Risk level	Microbial risk
0	No threat	No *E. coli* or Enterococci detected in previous 2 seasonal samples
1-3	Tolerable	*E. coli* or Enterococci detected of no more than 1 out of previous 2 seasonal samples taken and using counts 1 / 100ml.
4-6	Peripheral	*E. coli* or Enterococci detected of more than 1 out of previous 2 seasonal samples taken and counts 10 / 100ml.
7-10	Not tolerable	*E. coli* or Enterococci detected of more than 1 out of previous 2 seasonal samples taken and counts >10 / 100ml.

The WHO/UNICEF (2012) ON THE Toolkit for monitoring and evaluating household water treatment and safe storage programmes was used to determine the score and the intervention required, where 7-10 score is detected urgent intervention measures will be required while 4-6 require high and 1-3 is considered a low risk where low action is needed; and community should be informed on how to prepare their water to make it safe for consumption (WHO/UNICEF, 2012).

Conclusion

The review highlighted the need for provision of basic water service which is accessible, available, potable, affordable and sustainable. The importance of measuring basic water service delivery through indicators to benchmark WSA's performance was shown. Where one concept is not attained it could escalate the risks faced by the community in terms of their welfare. More emphasis was based on the need for WSA's on the set indicators that goes along with the concepts.

An analysis of these indicators was done based on what was set internationally and in SA water and sanitation policy of 1994. Relevant policy documents and legislations available in SA were also outlined. An equation based on the water quantity accessed and distance travelled by the household was developed to assist on the WSA's to measure the level of services provided to its communities. The outcomes are measured against the quantity and quality of water provided based on the analysis done as well as the level of risks that could be incurred by such community. However the indicators that are benchmarked leave some elements that are important to be included in the water service indicators. However, the review indicated the importance of using water service indicators as WSA's performance monitor and measurable outcome of the service provided to communities. To assess its performance based on the scores developed, WSA's could measure its performance and the level of score will determine where interventions need to be taken. That will trigger the need to make analysis on the challenges that impact the service rendered. If WSA's have a way of measuring sustainable water service delivery; more effort could be done to correct the situation and compliance to the policy. The equation and scores outlined could be used as a better method of quantifying the level of service to WSA's. It should be noted that this review did not look at the financial or economic issues, measurement of right to water access and in depth analyses in terms of public health outcomes; only risk-base analyses was done. There are number of ways that were proposed to quantify water service level but were not tested.

Recommendations

The following are recommendations based on this review;

- More studies that provide evidence on the beneficial and consequences of the indicators on availability and accessibility need to be done.
- Rapid method to calculate water quantity available and accessibility per capita need to be tested.
- Scores on availability and accessibility are required for proper measurements.
- There is a need to conduct further studies on water service indicators and risks that might be incurred by the communities as outlined both in SA and internationally
- SA water indicators need to be reviewed

- Household water safety policy on water treatment and storage should be considered and aligned with water and sanitation policy.

References

African National Congress (1994), *African National Congress Reconstruction and Development programme. A Policy Framework,* Johannesburg: Umanyano Publications.

Atusinguza, F. & Egbuna, C. (2012), 'A microbiological risk assessment of a private water supply in Southeast England: Implication for future policy', in *Journal of Life Science and Biomedicine,* 3: 40-51.

Bartram, J. (2009), *Water safety plan manual: step-by-step risk management for drinking-water suppliers*, Geneva: World Health Organization.

Boone, C., Glick, P. & Sahn, D. (2011), 'Household water supply choice and time allocated to water collection: Evidence from Madagascar', in *Journal of Development Studies,* 47: 1826-1850.

Bradley, D. J. & Bartram, D. K. (2013), 'Domestic water and sanitation as water security: monitoring, concepts and strategy', *Philosophical Transactions of the Royal Society A: Mathematical, Physical and Engineering Sciences,* 371, 20120420.

Clasen, T. (2010), 'Household water treatment and the mellennium development goals: keeping the focus on health', in *Environmental Science and Technology*, 4.

Crow, B., Davies, J., Paterson, S. & Miles, J. (2013), 'Using GPS and recall to understand water collection in Kenyan informal settlements', in *Water International,* 38: 43-60.

Dar, O. A. & Khan, M. S. (2011), 'Millennium development goals and the water target: details, definitions and debate', in *Tropical Medicine & International Health,* 16: 540-544.

Davison, A., Howard, G., Stevens, M., Callan, P., Fewtrell, L., Deere, D. & Bartram, J. (2005), *Water safety plans,* Geneva: World Health Organization.

De Coning, C. & Sherwill, T. (2004), *An assessment of the water policy process in South Africa (1994 to 2003),* Pretoria, South Africa: Water Research Commission Pretoria.

Department of Water Affairs (1994), *Water supply and sanitation policy*, Cape Town, South Africa.

Department of Water Affairs (1998), *Quality of domestic water supplies volume 1: Assessment Guide,* Pretoria, South Africa: Water Research Commission.

Department of Water Affairs (2002), *Free Basic Water Implementation GuidelinesFree Basic Water Implementation Strategy*, Pretoria, South Africa: Department of Water Affairs.

Department of Water Affairs (2005), 'Drinking water quality regulation strategy', *In:* Affairs, D. O. W. (ed.). Pretoria, South Africa: Department of Water Affairs.

Department of Water Affairs (2009), *Blue Drop Report,* Pretoria, South Africa: Department of Water Affairs.

Department of Water Affairs (2010), *National water services regulation strategy*, Pretoria, South Africa: Department of Water Affairs.

Department of Water Affairs (2010),. *Department of Water Affairs Annual Report 2009/2010*. Pretoria, South Africa.

DWAF (1994), *Water supply and sanitation policy*, Cape Town, South Africa.

Evans, B., Bartram, J., Hunter, P., Rhoderick Williams, A., Geere, J., Majuru, B., Bates, L., Fisher, M., Overbo, A. & Schmidt, W.-P. (2013), *Public Health and Social Benefits of at-house Water Supplies,* The Final Report, 21 June 2013, Leeds University, UK.

Gelting, R. C. (2009), *Water Safety Plan CDC's Role* [on line]. A. National Health Institute, USA.

Hay, R., Hay, P., Mlisa, A., Blake, D., Imrie, S. & Goldberg, K. (2012), *A risk-based methodology to assess social vulnerability in the context of water infrastructure,* Pretoria, South Africa: Water Research Commission.

Hope, R. (2006), 'Evaluating water policy scenarios against the priorities of the rural poor', in *World Development,* 34: 167-179.

Hosking, S. G. & Jacoby, K. T. (2013), *Trends in the insight into the growing South African Municipal water service delivery problem*, Pretoria, South Africa: Water research commission.

Howard, G. & Bartram, J. (2003), *Domestic water quantity, service level, and health,* Genever: World Health Organization.

Hunter, P., Macdonald, A. & Carter, R. (2010), 'Water supply and health',in *PLoS medicine,* 7**,** e1000361.

Hunter, P., Pond, K., Jagals, P. & Cameron, J. (2009a), 'An assessment of the costs and benefits of interventions aimed at improving rural community water supplies in developed countries', in *Science of the Total Environment* 407**,** 5.

Hunter, P., Zmirou-Navier, D. & Hartemann, P. (2009b), 'Estimating the impact on health of poor reliability of drinking water interventions in developing countries', in *Science of the Total Environment,* 407**,** 4.

Jagals, P. (2006), 'Does improved access to water supply by rural households enhance the concept of safe water at the point of use? A case study from deep rural South Africa', in *Water Science and Technology,* 54**:** 8.

Künzle, R. & Morgenroth, E. (2011), *Household drinking-water quality in the Kenyan Rift Valley,* Masters Thesis, Swiss Federal Institute of Technology, Zurich.

Majuru, B., Jagals, P. & Hunter, P. (2012), 'Assessing rural small community water supply in Limpopo, South Africa: Water service benchmarks and reliability', in *Science of the Total Environment,* 435**:** 479-486.

Mansour, S. A. E. A. (2011), *Developing GIS analysis techniques for the measurement of safe drinking water access,* PhD Thesis, University of Southampton, UK.

Mellor, J. E., Smith, J. A., Learmonth, G. P., Netshandama, V. O. & Dillingham, R. A. (2012), 'Modeling the complexities of water, hygiene, and health in Limpopo Province, South Africa', in *Environmental science & technology,* 46: 13512-13520.

Mokoena, M. M. & Jagals, P. (2009), *The effect of water-supply service delivery on the risk of infection posed by water in household containers,* Dept Environmental Health, Faculty of Science, Tshwane University of Technology, Pretoria. Available at: http://www.ewisa.co.za/literature/files/80_33%20Mokoena.pdf

Moriarty, P., Batchelor, C., Fonseca, C., Klutse, A., Naafs, A., Nyarko, K., Pezon, C., Potter, A., Reddy, R. & Snehalatha, M. (2010), *Ladders for assessing and costing water service delivery*, IRC International Water and Sanitation Centre.

Municipal Structures Act (1997), *Local Government: Municipal Structures Act 117 of 1997*,

Pretoria, South Africa: SA government Printers.

National Water Act. (1998), 'National Water Act No.36 of 1998', *In:* AFFAIRS, D. O. W. (ed.). Pretoria, South Africa: SA Government, Printers.

Nnaji, C. C., Eluwa, C. & Nwoji, C. (2013), 'Dynamics of domestic water supply and consumption in a semi-urban Nigerian city', in *Habitat International,* 40: 127-135.

Peter, G. (2010), 'Impact of rural water projects on hygienic behaviour in Swaziland', in *Physics and Chemistry of the Earth, Parts A/B/C,* 35: 772-779.

Pickering, A. J. & Davis, J. (2012), 'Freshwater availability and water fetching distance affect child health in sub-Saharan Africa', *Environmental Science & Technology,* 46: 2391-2397.

Prüss-Üstün, A., Bos, R., Gore, F. & Bartram, J. (2008), *Safer water, better health: costs, benefits and sustainability of interventions to protect and promote health,* Geneve: World Health Organization.

Risebro, H. L., Breton, L., Aird, H., Hooper, A. & Hunter, P. R. (2012), 'Contaminated small drinking water supplies and risk of infectious intestinal disease: a prospective cohort study', *plos One,* 7, e42762.

SA Constitution Act 108. (1996), *Constitution of the Republic of South Africa, No 108 of 1996,* Pretoria, South Africa: Government Printers.

SA Water Service Act 108. (1997), *Republic of South Africa Water Service Act, 108 of 1997*, Pretoria, South Africa: Government Printers.

Smith, J. (2010), 'How much water is enough? Domestic metered water consumption and free basic water volumes: The case of Eastwood, Pietermaritzburg', in *Water SA,* 36: 595-606.

Sobsey, M. (2002), *Managing water in the home: accelerated health gains from improved water supply,* Geneva.

South African Bureau of Standard (2006), *South African National Standard (SANS) 241: 2006. Drinking water standard,* Pretoria, South Africa, Standards South Africa.

Sphere Project (2004), Humanitarian Charter and Minimum Standards in Disaster Response. *Minimum Standards in Water Supply, Sanitation and Hygiene Promotion.* Geneva, Switzerland.

Tambekar, D. H., Gulhane, S. R., Jaisingkar, R. S., Wangikar, M. S., Banginwar, Y. S. & Mogarekar, M. R. (2008), 'Household Water management: A systematic study of bacteriological contamination between source and point-of-use', in *American-Eurasian Journal of Agriculture and Environmental Science,* 3: 241-246.

Tapela, B. N. (2012), *Social water scarcity and water use*, Pretoria, South Africa: Water Research Commission.

Taulo, S., Wetlesen, A., Abrahamsen, R., Mkakosya, R. & Kululanga, G. (2008), 'Microbiological quality of water, associated management practices and risks at source, transport and storage points in a rural community of Lungwena, Malawi', in *Afr. J. Microbiol. Res,* 7,: 131-137.

United Nations (2013a), *The Millennium Development Goals Report*, New York.

United Nations (2013b), The equitable access score-card, *Supporting policy processes to achieve the human right to water and sanitation,* United Nations, Geneva, Switzerland.

Wang, X. & Hunter, P. R. (2010), 'A systematic review and meta-analysis of the association between self-reported diarrheal disease and distance from home to water source', in *The American journal of tropical medicine and hygiene,* 83: 582.

Wate, S. R. (2012), 'An Overview of Policies Impacting Water Quality and Governance in India', in *International Journal of Water Resources Development,* 28: 265-279.

Water Aid (2009), *Management for sustainability: Practical lessons from three studies on the management of rural water supply schemes,* Dar es Salaam, Tanzania.

Water Research Commission (2012), *Water Research Commission Draft Strategic Plan 2012/13 – 2016/17*, Pretoria, South Africa: Water Research Commission.

WHO (2011), *Guideline for Drinking Water Quality*, Geneva: World Health Organization.

WHO (2008), *Guidelines for Drinking-water Quality,* Geneva: World Health Organization.

WHO/UNICEF (2008), *Joint monitoring Programme for water and Sanitation: Progress on sanitation and drinking water,* Geneva, Switzerland.

WHO/UNICEF (2012), *Progress on Drinking Water and Sanitation 2012 Update,* United States of America.

WHO Library Cataloguing.

WHO/UNICEF (2012), *A toolkit for monitoring and evaluating household water treatment and safe storage programmes*, Geneva, Switzerland.

Chapter 13

Post Scriptum

Water and Sanitation for Green Innovative Economic Development of Hope

Mammo Muchie & Angathevar Baskaran

There are a number of challenges related to water and sanitation that require collaboration globally to address them. A key challenge is that water exists unevenly globally being abundant in some areas and scarce in other areas. The way the world is geographacally parceled with uneven distribution of water resources creates problems such as water scarcity. The existing climate change risk can exacerbate the water scarcity dilemma leading to reduction in the Gross Domestic Product which in turn can lead to migration and domestic strife and conflict. As the world population is growing and urbanisation is expanding, a gap between water supply and demand can widen making it difficult to find a reasonable solution. The supply of water can decrease owing to the erratic climatic impact along with growing demands by the rising number of the world population.

There is a need to find ways to maintain the water that is abundant and share with those areas where water scarcity is in short supply. The areas of the world where there are deserts like Sahara and Sahel in Africa where there is water scarcity need to create hydrowater technology to convert the deseret into a green zone by finding scientific and engineering resources to convert the energy to increase water supply and reduce water scarcity. If the regions fail to manage their water resources, they will run into health and economic development quagmire creating insecurity, migration and conflict. Climatic changes and conditions that create drought and floods can exacerbate the political and economic development pathways for those countries that cannot cope with the management of the supply and demand of water. How to discover ways to manage water to make a country's economy innovative and green at this time of the 4th industrial revolution is very critical.

As water is considered a human right, equally food is also a human right. Water for agriculture to create productivity for food security is a truly pivotal policy that cannot be put aside. It should serve as a central strategy for applying available water and finding even efficiently better water resources to provide food for all the people in a given economy particularly in regions where there is geographically water scarcity. There should be appropriate forcasting and foresight to avoid inefficient water use with forward and onward anticipation of both the risks and benefits in the planning of water resource use and application.

Water abundant regions should work to organise with incentives the infrastructure to make all their neigbours and themselves in collaboration to deal effectively and efficiently with climate change risks by mobilising investment to sustain secure water supply resources. There can be a world trade in accessing clean water supply and sanitation and by using hydrology. There can also be water companies with global reach that can facilitate virtual water movement across the world.There is a need to address not just technology and infrastructure but global water governance to translate into practice the conceptual framing of water as a human right. The UN in its World Water Development Report has addressed the water governance dimension along with all the other necessary needs such as human capacity and available financial resources but also water and natural resources.

Water security will remain a big challenge despite the good news of many countries achieving the MDG goals related to water. The existing mode of economic growth with population also growing is likely to put heavy burden in meeting the clean water and sanitation standard that can serve to define the human rights recognition and application. If the current economic and population growth trends continue the likelihood the prediction is that there will be shortfalls between growing demand and the supply of water in the coming decades. Prediction is that world population will grow to 9 billion and that will put pressure to produce adequate food and water. The need to use water for agriculture to feed so many people will demand water that may not be available everywhere on demand.It is not for agriculture only, but water is also needed for hydroelectricity generation. The prediction is that there will be more people who live in conditions of absolute water scarcity that will affect food security and reliable electricity provisions. This will exacerbate sanitation which was one of the most off-track MDG goals outcomes globally. It means sanitation too can go worse and may even remain off-track even in the SDGs by 2030. The risk is high that the world may be off-track rather than being on-track to fulfill the SDG goals by providing food , water and sanitation in an environment where people reside in livable urban settlements and residences with education and human development equipped with the provisions of energy and climate security. If the world is going to realise on time the SDGs, what is clearly evident is the fact that management of water resources to ensure access to reliable water and sanitation services is a primary goal that all stake-holders should decide and begin to address without any delay.

There is a need to promote renewable, alternative or green energy. Historicaly hydropower has been the source of electricity and energy. Hydroelectric power is said to be one of the oldest sources of electricity. Today hydropower produces the world's largest source of renewable energy and it is also said to be accounting for a fifth of global electricity, which means water is not only for drinking or promoting agriculture to provide food security but also for harnessing electricity. What needs a new wave of innovations is not only the harnessing of water to facilitate the provision of electricity, but there is a need to make a pardigm shift from economics as it is to promote the economics of hope. There is a need for global collaboration to reduce the global average temperature based on the Paris agreement on Climate Change. This means a new economics where renewable energy and hydropower drive the global climate are essential. A new green, innovative, sustainable economics of hope is needed if water and sanitation are to be an integral part of the creation a new, safe and healthy environment where the wellbeing of people and nature become the priority of priorties to realise the goal of social and economic transformation and development.

Notes on Contributors

Mammo Muchie

DST/NRF SARChI Professor (Innovation & Development), Tshwane University of Technology, South Africa; Technology and Management Centre for Development (TMCD), Oxford University, UK; Associate Faculty Professor, Sussex University, UK; University of Gondar, Arsi University & Adama Science and Technology University (ASTU), Ethiopia. Email: MuchieM@tut.ac.za

Angathevar Baskaran

Associate Professor, Department of Development Studies, Faculty of Economics and Administration, University of Malaya, Malaysia; Senior Research Associate of SARChI (Innovation & Development), Tshwane University of Technology, Pretoria, South Africa. Email: baskaran@um.edu.my & anga_bas@yahoo.co.uk

Oluwakemi S. Babatunde

Department of Sociology, Landmark University, PMB 1001, OmuAran, Kwara State, Nigeria. Email: babatundeshade.k@gmail.com

Olawale O. Olanrewaju

School of Civil and Environmental Engineering, University of the Witwatersrand, Johannesburg. South Africa. Department of Agricultural Engineering, Federal University of Technology, Akure, Nigeria. Email: Olawale.Olanrewaju@students.wits.ac.za.

James R. Adewumi

School of Civil and Environmental Engineering, University of the Witwatersrand, Johannesburg. South Africa.Department of Civil Engineering, Federal University of Technology, Akure, Nigeria. Email: adrotimi2003@yahoo.com.

Emmanuel M. Akpabio

Department of Geography and Regional Planning, University of Uyo, P. O. Box 4223, Uyo, Akwa Ibom State, Nigeria. Email: emakpabio@yahoo.com

Rasheed A. Adeleke

School of Environmental Sciences and Development: Microbiology North-West University: Potchefstroom campus, Private Bag X6001, Potchefstroom, 2520, South Africa. Email:r_adeleke@yahoo.com; 20116799@nwu.ac.za.

Cornelius C. Bezuidenhout

School of Environmental Sciences and Development: Microbiology,North-West University, Potchefstroom Campus, Private Bag X6001, Potchefstroom, 2520, South Africa. Email: Carlos.Bezuidenhout@nwu.ac.za.

Oghenerobor B. Akpor

Institute for Economic Research on Innovation, Tshwane University of Technology, 159 Skinner Street, Pretoria 0001, South Africa. Email: AkporBO@tut.ac.za

Maxwell K. Boakye

Department of Environmental Management, Tshwane University of Technology, Pretoria 0001, South Africa. Email: maxwell_boakye@yahoo.com

Bilainu O. Oboirien

CSIR Materials Science and Manufacturing, PO Box, 395, Pretoria 0001, South Africa. Email: boboirien@csir.co.za

Nwankwoala, H.O.

Department of Geology, University of Port Harcourt, Nigeria. E-mail: nwankwoala_ho@yahoo.com; hyci2002@yahoo.com

Udom, G. J.

Department of Geology, University of Port Harcourt, Nigeria.

Segun Oshewolo

Department of Political Science, Landmark University, Omuaran, Nigeria. E-mail: segunoshewolo@yahoo.com

Matodzi M Mokoena

Department of Environmental Health, Tshwane University of Technology, Private Bag X680, Pretoria, 0001, Republic of South Africa.

Murembiwa S Mukhola

Deputy Vice-Chancellor: Teaching, Learning and Technology (Acting), Tshwane University of Technology, Private Bag X 680, Pretoria, 0001, Republic of South Africa, Email: Mukholams@tut.ac.za

Lutendo S Mudau

Tshwane University of Technology, Environmental Health Department Pretoria, Republic of South Africa, Email: mudauls@tut.ac.za

Paul R Hunter

University of East Anglia, Norwich School of Medicine, Norwich, NR4 7TJ, United Kingdom, Email: Paul.hunter@uea.ac.uk

Index

A

B

C

D

E

F

G

H

I

J

K

N

O

P

Q

R

T

Y